Celiac Disease

Edited by Jianyuan Chai

Published in London, United Kingdom

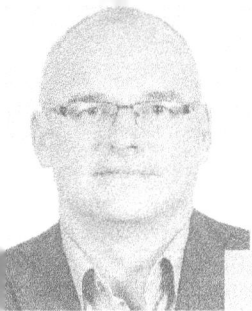
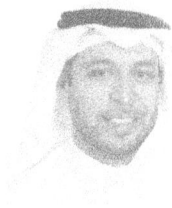
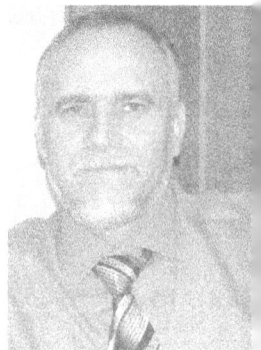
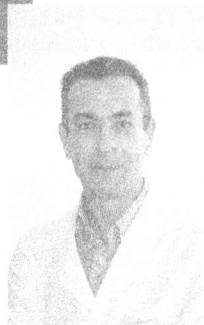
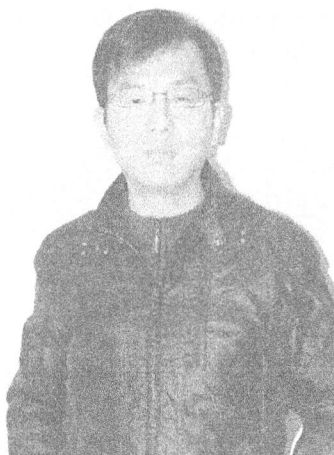
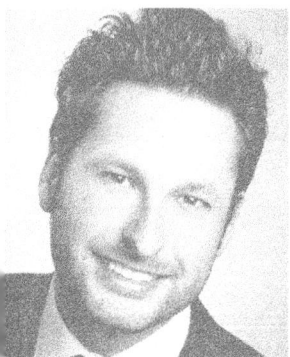
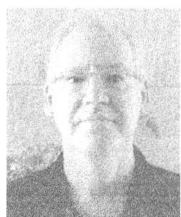

IntechOpen

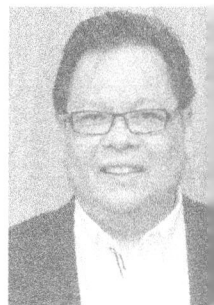
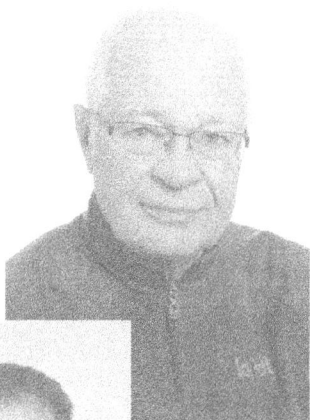
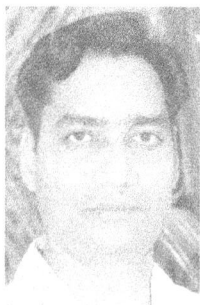
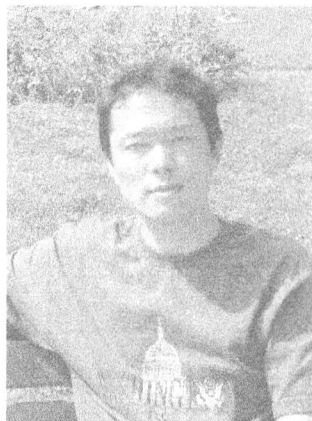
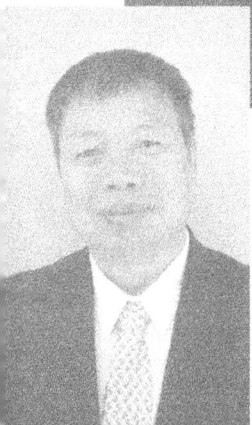
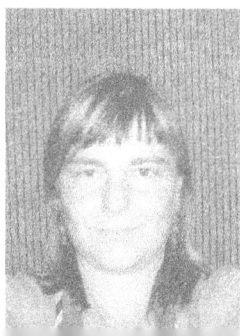

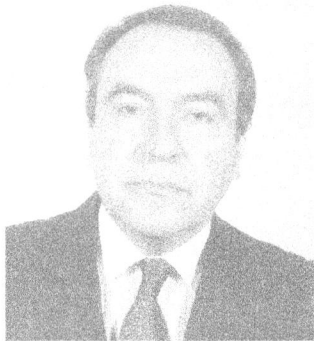

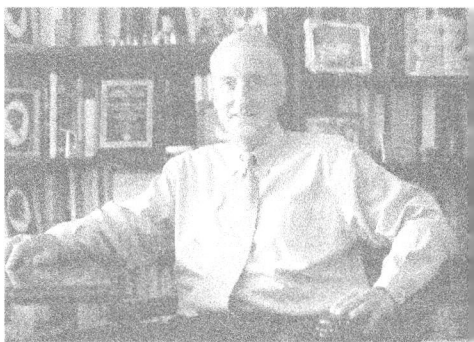

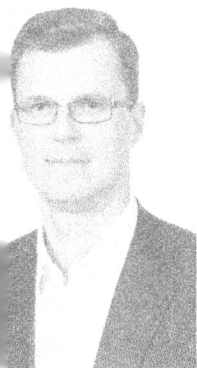

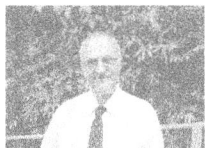

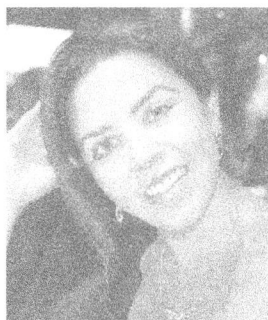

Supporting open minds since 2005

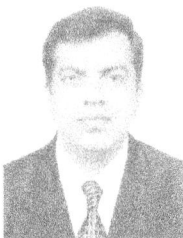

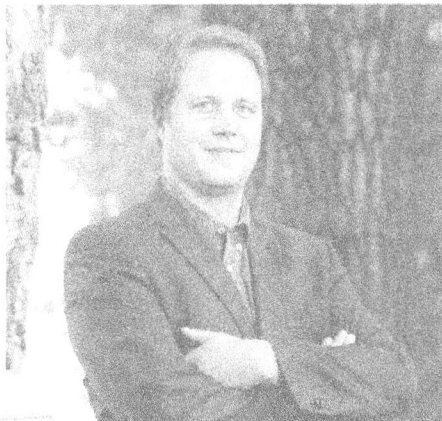

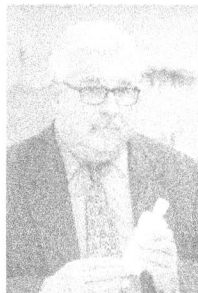

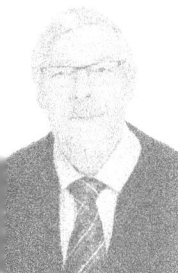

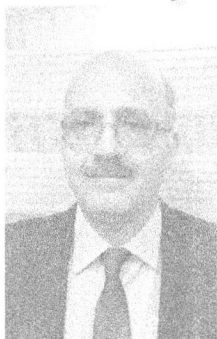

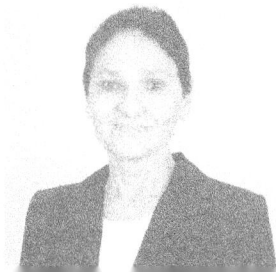

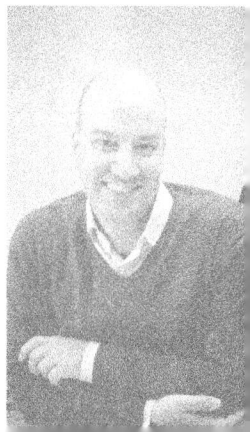

Celiac Disease
http://dx.doi.org/10.5772/intechopen.87265
Edited by Jianyuan Chai

Contributors
Paul J. Ciclitira, Isabel Torres, Miguel Ángel López Casado, Pedro Lorite, Federica Gualandris, Laura Castellani, Anna Falanga, Babatunde Olawoye, Oseni Kadiri, Oladapo Fisoye Fagbohun, Timilehin David Oluwajuyitan, Jianyuan Chai, Teresa Palomeque, Alastair Forbes

Notice
Statements and opinions expressed in the chapters are these of the individual contributors and not necessarily those of the editors or publisher. No responsibility is accepted for the accuracy of information contained in the published chapters. The publisher assumes no responsibility for any damage or injury to persons or property arising out of the use of any materials, instructions, methods or ideas contained in the book.

First published in London, United Kingdom, 2021 by IntechOpen
IntechOpen is the global imprint of INTECHOPEN LIMITED, registered in England and Wales, registration number: 11086078, 5 Princes Gate Court, London, SW7 2QJ, United Kingdom
Printed in Croatia

British Library Cataloguing-in-Publication Data
A catalogue record for this book is available from the British Library

Additional hard and PDF copies can be obtained from orders@intechopen.com

Celiac Disease
Edited by Jianyuan Chai
p. cm.
Print ISBN 978-1-83962-535-0
Online ISBN 978-1-83962-536-7
eBook (PDF) ISBN 978-1-83962-537-4

We are IntechOpen,
the world's leading publisher of
Open Access books
Built by scientists, for scientists

5,300+
Open access books available

130,000+
International authors and editors

155M+
Downloads

Our authors are among the

156
Countries delivered to

Top 1%
most cited scientists

12.2%
Contributors from top 500 universities

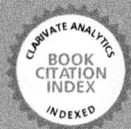

Interested in publishing with us?
Contact book.department@intechopen.com

Numbers displayed above are based on latest data collected.
For more information visit www.intechopen.com

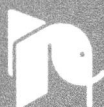

Meet the editor

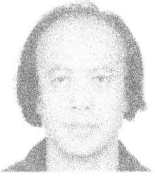

Dr. Jianyuan Chai received his Ph.D. in Biology from the City University of New York in 1998 and completed his postdoctoral training at Harvard University in 2001. He served the Department of Veterans Affairs of the United States as a Principal Investigator from 2002 to 2016, in affiliation with the School of Medicine, University of California, Irvine. Currently, he is a professor at Baotou Medical College, Inner Mongolia University of Science and Technology. He has published dozens of research articles on various subjects including zoology, cardiovascular biology, gastroenterology, and cancer biology. He has been a member of AGA, AHA, ASBMB, and several other professional organizations. He has also served on the editorial boards of multiple journals.

Contents

Preface

Celiac disease is a common autoimmune disorder triggered by eating gluten, a protein found in wheat, rye, and barley. At least 1% of the current world population is affected by this disease. Despite many years of effort, the pathogenesis of celiac disease is still not understood completely. We do know that all celiac disease patients have either the DQ2 or DQ8 gene, but only 1%-3% of these individuals develop the disease. Obviously, other factors must be involved. Over the years, many factors have been investigated for their possible contributions to the onset of celiac disease, including some unusual ones like age, socioeconomic status, education level, and so on; however, none of these is sufficient to solve the puzzle.

This book contains five chapters, each of which covers an important aspect of celiac disease. Following the Introductory chapter which is Chapter 1, in the second chapter Gualandris et al. analyze the primary contributor to celiac, the DQ2 gene. They examine its role in celiac disease as well as its connections with other abnormalities, such as diabetes, irritable bowel syndrome (IBS), inflammatory bowel disease (IBD), HIV, autism, and multiple sclerosis. In Chapter 3, Torres et al. discuss the immune checkpoints of IDO, HLA-G, CTLA, and PD1, providing directions for new therapeutic options. In Chapter 4, Ciclitira and Forbes present a focused review on refractory celiac disease, including how it occurs, its clinical features, how it is diagnosed and treated, and possible complications. In Chapter 5, Olawoye et al. discuss the current status of the gluten-free diet, the only recognized solution for celiac disease thus far.

Celiac disease is not just a health issue. It is also an economic one that has placed a tremendous burden on the economies of many countries. For instance, the United States spent $2.3 billion in 2019 on gluten-free food products. This budget could reach $4.5 billion by 2027. The United Kingdom invested £426 million in this market in 2018 and plans to increase this investment by 40% by 2030. If we can discover other ways to eliminate celiac disease, it would be a big lift to the world economy. This book is our effort towards this goal.

Jianyuan Chai
Inner Mongolia Institute of Digestive Diseases,
Baotou Medical College,
Inner Mongolia University of Science and Technology,
Baotou, China

Chapter 1

Introductory Chapter: Celiac Disease - Now and Then

Jianyuan Chai

1. Introduction

   Celiac disease, in one sentence, can probably be defined as a complex autoimmune disorder triggered by gluten ingestion in people carrying the HLA-DQ2 or HLA-DQ8 gene. The most common symptom associated with the disease is diarrhea after eating gluten-containing food, such as wheat, rye, or barley products. The earliest documentation about the celiac disease can be traced back to the 2nd century AD and it was written by a Greek physician named Aretaeus the Cappadocian [1]. He used the Greek word "koiliakos" or "coeliacs" to call it, meaning abdomen discomfort. He said in English translation: "If the stomach be irretentive of food and if it passes through undigested and crude, and nothing ascends into the body, we call such persons coeliacs". He also identified the connection between the illness and eating bread and learned that fasting was helpful to reduce the symptoms. This knowledge was elaborated 1700 years later by a British doctor, Samuel Jones Gee, in his lecture entitled "On the Celiac Affection" [2]. He revealed the fact that celiac disease could affect not only children but also adults, but mostly children under 5 years old. If the patient must eat bread, he suggested, "Bread cut thin and well toasted on both sides … But if the patient can be cured at all, it must be by means of diet". This is consistent with our knowledge today. A more interesting description about the celiac disease was found in the three lectures given by Professor George F. Still at the Royal College of Physicians of London [3], who vividly pictured his observation of the sick children: "What appears to be an infant little more than 12 months old … it is at least a year or two older, perhaps three or four years older, than its appearance would suggest". Now we know that this is due to malnutrition associated with such eating disorders. Another important discovery was made by Dicke, a Dutch pediatrician, who noticed that celiac disease almost vanished in the Netherlands during World War II when bread was on a serious scarcity, but it came back quickly when the Swedish airplanes dropped bread to the region. Later, he figured out that it was gluten that made people sick [4]. Starting from the mid-20th century, people have been developing various endoscopic tools to reach into the duodenum or even further down into the small intestine to obtain tissue samples for pathological analysis. This technology significantly accelerated our understanding of the pathogenesis of the celiac disease [5]. Later on, gluten antibodies were discovered in patients with celiac disease and their diagnostic value was soon recognized in the medical community [6]. This work built the foundation for serological detection of celiac disease today. From the 70s, people started to look for the possible genetic reasons for celiac disease, and soon a connection with HLA-DQ2 and HLA-DQ8 expression was found [7, 8]. After the 90s, our current concept of celiac disease was gradually formed: this is an autoimmune disorder that can be triggered by gluten ingestion in people with a DQ2 or DQ8 genetic background.

Looking back the history, our understanding of celiac disease has experienced such path: presentations of the disease (ancient time till 19th century) – identification of gluten as the cause (mid-20th century) – pathology of the disease (the 50-the 60s) – immunology of the disease (the 60–70s) – genetics of the disease (the 70–80s) – current concept of the disease (after the 90s).

2. Pathogenesis of celiac disease

Gluten is a common name for the viscoelastic proteins present in various grains, such as gliadin from wheat, hordein from barley, and secaline from rye. The main amino acids of these proteins are glutamine and proline (or collectively called prolamine), which makes them resistant to proteolytic enzymes of the human gut. Using gliadin as an example, gliadin contains 35% glutamine and 15% proline and can only be broken down to oligopeptides of 20–50 amino acids in the human intestine. For the majority of people, these peptides remain in the lumen of the intestine and eventually are expelled out from the body, but for those individuals who carry HLA-DQ2/DQ8 genes, they can bind to the chemokine receptor CXCR3 on the intestinal epithelial cells to induce zonulin overexpression. Zonulin in structure is similar to the zona occludens toxin from *Vibrio cholera* and has the function to disassemble the tight junctions between epithelial cells via protease activated receptor 2/EGFR pathway. This allows the half-digested gluten peptides to pass through the mucosal barrier and reach the lamina propria [9]. Gluten peptides can also reach the lamina propria through the epithelial cells using IgA/CD71 channels. Once getting into the lamina propria, these peptides are deamidated by tissue transglutaminase 2 (tTG2), converting glutamine to glutamate, which makes them easier to be taken up by HLA-DQ2 and –DQ8 bearing antigen-presenting cells. This triggers the generation of gluten-specific CD4+ T lymphocytes [10]. Upon gluten stimulation, these gluten-specific T cells start to produce a lot of pro-inflammatory cytokines, including interleukin (IL)-15, IL-21, and interferon-γ. IL-15 stimulates CD8+ T cells to migrate to the epithelial layer to attack the epithelial cells, causing villous atrophy, a hallmark of celiac disease [11]. Gluten-specific T cells also promote the activation of B cells, which develop into plasma cells, producing the autoantibodies against tTG2, which is used nowadays as the biomarker in serological tests for celiac disease [12].

Although all of the celiac disease patients are either DQ2 or DQ8 positive, only 1–3% of the people with such genetic background develop the disease [13, 14], indicating that other factors must be involved. Microbial infection in the duodenum has been postulated to play a role. For instance, *Pseudomonas aeruginosa*, a bacteria that is commonly found in the duodenum of celiac disease patients, produces elastases that can degrade the gluten into highly immunogenic peptides [15]. Other factors that have been investigated for their possible contributions to the onset of celiac disease include (1) time and amount of gluten consumption in infants [16–18], (2) virus infection [19, 20], (3) *H. pylori* eradication [21, 22], (4) maternal gluten consumption [23], (5) maternal C-section [24–26], (6) maternal iron deficiency [27, 28], (7) summer birth [29–31], (8) maternal high education [32], (9) maternal non-smoking [33], (10) high socio-economic status [34, 35], (11) geographic locations [36–38], (12) Vitamin D deficiency [39], (13) antibiotic use in childhood [40], and (14) PPI use [41]. However, none of these factors are sufficient to solve the puzzle completely. It seems that each one of these factors plays a part but they (at least some of them) must work together to trigger the intestinal allergy to gluten and the subsequent clinical manifestations of celiac disease.

While many years of effort has been made, the pathogenesis of celiac disease still remains as a mystery today.

3. Current therapeutic strategies for celiac disease

Since celiac disease is troubling at least 1% of the world population, people have been actively searching for therapeutic solutions to control the disease. The effort has been focusing on each key component in the entire pathogenic process, which can be classified into the following five categories.

3.1 Reduction of gluten immunogenicity

The simplest way that one can think of to cure celiac disease is to stop eating all gluten-containing food. Without the trigger, the disease of course will never occur. Believe it or not, this is the most effective method thus far to treat celiac disease – a gluten-free diet. However, wheat products have been the main component of our daily meals for thousands of years, not only for the Western world but also for the Orientals. The only difference between the western bread and the eastern bread is that the former is baked and the latter is steamed. Quitting such a lifestyle for most people is hard to do. For this reason, scientists have been trying to engineer wheat genetically so that it will produce flour containing less or not all gluten without losing much of the original gastronomic properties. Unfortunately, this has not been very successful so far [42, 43].

3.2 Prevention of gluten degradation

The idea is to use synthetic polymers or specific antibodies to sequester gluten in the gut so that it would not be degraded into an immunogen. BL-7010 is such a polymer. *In vitro* analyses as well as animal studies all showed promising results, including no toxicity [44], gluten selectivity [45], and villous protection [46]. Now its clinical trials are underway. Using antibodies to seize gluten in the intestine has also gained encouraging results. AGY is an IgY antibody generated from chicken eggs against gluten. Taking AGY capsules has been shown capable to reduce gliadin absorption from 42.8% to 0.7% in an animal study [47]. A clinical trial with AGY also obtained effectiveness [48].

3.3 Prevention of gluten peptides entering intestinal mucosa

The next target is intestinal epithelial integrity. The majority of gluten peptides get to the lamina propria through para-cellular space, which is sealed by tight junctions in healthy individuals. Overexpression of zonulin triggered by gluten stimulation in DQ2/DQ8 carriers causes a collapse of the tight junctions. Therefore, if mucosal permeability is restricted, gluten peptides will largely remain in the intestinal lumen. Larazotide acetate is an octa-peptide developed against zonulin. Phase I and II clinical trials all showed substantial improvement in clinical symptoms, although some patients had some minor side-effect, such as headache and urinary infections [49–52].

3.4 Inhibition of tissue transglutaminase

As mentioned above, the immunogenicity of gluten peptides in celiac disease patients is largely dependent on their deamidation by tTG-2. Therefore, inhibition of tTG-2 activity would reduce the amount of immunogen production. Because tTG-2 activation also contributes to several other diseases, such as Parkinson's, Alzheimer's, Huntington's, and even some cancers, a great effort has been put in to develop tTG-2 inhibitors. An animal study has shown some encouraging results using this strategy in the treatment of celiac disease. A phase II clinical trial has been initiated.

3.5 Prevention of immune reaction

Celiac disease is an autoimmune disorder. The therapeutic strategies discussed above all intend to stop gluten from becoming an immunogen. The last approach is targeting the immune reaction assuming the four strategies above all failed. This includes using chemical blockers to mask the active sites of DQ2, using immunodominant gluten peptides to vaccinate DQ2/DQ8 carriers, transplanting special bacteria that are capable to produce nontoxic gluten in the human gut, using steroids, etc. Many such products will be out soon.

Author details

Jianyuan Chai
Inner Mongolia Institute of Digestive Diseases, The Second Affiliated Hospital of Baotou Medical College, Inner Mongolia University of Science and Technology, Baotou, China

*Address all correspondence to: jianyuan.chai@gmail.com

IntechOpen

References

[1] Adams F. The extant works of Aretaeus the Cappadocian. London: London Sydenham Society. 1856: 350.

[2] Gee SJ. On the coeliac affection. St. Bartholomew's Report. 1888; 24: 17-20.

[3] Still CF. The Lumleian Lectures on coeliac disease. Lancet. 1918; ii: 163-6, 193-7, 227-9.

[4] Dicke WK, Weijers HA, Van de Kamer JH. Coeliac disease. II. The presence in wheat of a factor having a deleterious effect in cases of coeliac disease. Acta Paediatr. 1953; 42: 34-42.

[5] Paveley WF. From Aretaeus to Crosby: a history of coeliac disease. Br Med J. 1988; 297: 1646-1649.

[6] Berger E, Buergin-wolff A, Freudenberg E. Diagnostic value of the demonstration of gliadin antibodies in celiac disease. Klin Wochenschr. 1964; 42: 788-790.

[7] Falchuk ZM, Rogentine GN, Strober W. Predominance of histocompatibility antigen HL-A8 in patients with gluten-sensitive enteropathy. J Clin Invest. 1972; 51: 1602-1605.

[8] Solhein BG, Ek J, Thune PO, Baklien K, Bratlie A, Rankin B, Thoresen AB, Thorsby E. HLA antigens in dermatitis herpetiformis and celiac disease. Tissue Antigens. 1976; 7: 57-59.

[9] Schumann M, Siegmund B, Schulzke JD, Fromm M. Celiac disease: Role of the Epithelial Barrier. Cell. Mol. Gastroenterol. Hepatol. 2017; 3: 150-162.

[10] Ting YT, Dahal-Koirala S, Kim HSK, Qiao SW, Neumann RS, Lundin KEA, Petersen J, Reid HH, Sollid LM, Rossjohn J. A molecular basis for the T cell response in HLA-DQ2.2 mediated celiac disease. Proc. Natl. Acad. Sci. USA. 2020; 117: 3063-3073.

[11] Jabri B, Sollid LM. T Cells in Celiac Disease. J. Immunol. 2017; 198: 3005-3014.

[12] Høydahl LS, Richter L, Frick R, Snir O, Gunnarsen KS, Landsverk OJB, Iversen R, Jeliazkov JR, Gray JJ, Bergseng E, Foss S, Qiao SW, Lundin KEA, Jahnsen J, Jahnsen FL, Sandlie I, Sollid LM, Løset GÅ. Plasma Cells Are the Most Abundant Gluten Peptide MHC-expressing Cells in Inflamed Intestinal Tissues From Patients With Celiac Disease. Gastroenterology. 2019; 156: 1428-1439.e10.

[13] Sollid LM, Markussen G, Ek J, Gjerde H, Vartdal F, Thorsby E. Evidence for a primary association of celiac disease to a particular HLA-DQ alpha/beta heterodimer. J Exp Med. 1989; 169: 345-350.

[14] Yuan J, Zhou C, Gao J, Li J, Yu F, Lu J, Li X, Wang X, Tong P, Wu Z, Yang A, Yao Y, Nadif S, Shu H, Jiang X, Wu Y, Gilissen L, Chen H. Prevalence of celiac disease autoimmunity among adolescents and young adults in China. Clin Gastroenterol Hepatol. 2017; 15:1572-1579 e1.

[15] Comino I, Real A, de Lorenzo L, Cornell H, López-Casado MÁ, Barro F, Lorite P, Torres MI, Cebolla A, Sousa C. Diversity in oat potential immunogenicity: basis for the selection of oat varieties with no toxicity in coeliac disease. Gut. 2011; 60:915-922.

[16] Lionetti E, Castellaneta S, Francavilla R, Pulvirenti A, Tonutti E, Amarri S, Barbato M, Barbera C, Barera G, Bellantoni A, Castellano E, Guariso G, Limongelli MG, Pellegrino S, Polloni C, Ughi C, Zuin G, Fasano A, Catassi C; SIGENP (Italian Society of

Pediatric Gastroenterology, Hepatology, and Nutrition) Working Group on Weaning and CD Risk. Introduction of gluten, HLA status, and the risk of celiac disease in children. N Engl J Med. 2014; 371:1295-1303.

[17] Vriezinga SL, Auricchio R, Bravi E, Castillejo G, Chmielewska A, Crespo Escobar P, Kolaček S, Koletzko S, Korponay-Szabo IR, Mummert E, Polanco I, Putter H, Ribes-Koninckx C, Shamir R, Szajewska H, Werkstetter K, Greco L, Gyimesi J, Hartman C, Hogen Esch C, Hopman E, Ivarsson A, Koltai T, Koning F, Martinez-Ojinaga E, te Marvelde C, Pavic A, Romanos J, Stoopman E, Villanacci V, Wijmenga C, Troncone R, Mearin ML. Randomized feeding intervention in infants at high risk for celiac disease. N Engl J Med. 2014; 371:1304-15.

[18] Andrén Aronsson C, Lee HS, Koletzko S, Uusitalo U, Yang J, Virtanen SM, Liu E, Lernmark Å, Norris JM, Agardh D; TEDDY Study Group. Effects of gluten intake on risk of celiac disease: a case‑control study on a swedish birth cohort. Clin Gastroenterol Hepatol. 2016; 14:403-409 e3.

[19] Stene LC, Honeyman MC, Hoffenberg EJ, Haas JE, Sokol RJ, Emery L, Taki I, Norris JM, Erlich HA, Eisenbarth GS, Rewers M. Rotavirus infection frequency and risk of celiac disease autoimmunity in early childhood: a longitudinal study. Am J Gastroenterol. 2006; 101:2333-2340.

[20] Bouziat R, Hinterleitner R, Brown JJ, Stencel-Baerenwald JE, Ikizler M, Mayassi T, Meisel M, Kim SM, Discepolo V, Pruijssers AJ, Ernest JD, Iskarpatyoti JA, Costes LM, Lawrence I, Palanski BA, Varma M, Zurenski MA, Khomandiak S, McAllister N, Aravamudhan P, Boehme KW, Hu F, Samsom JN, Reinecker HC, Kupfer SS, Guandalini S, Semrad CE, Abadie V,

Khosla C, Barreiro LB, Xavier RJ, Ng A, Dermody TS, Jabri B. Reovirus infection triggers inflammatory responses to dietary antigens and development of celiac disease. Science 2017; 356:44-50.

[21] Dore MP, Salis R, Loria MF, Villanacci V, Bassotti G, Pes GM. Helicobacter pylori infection and occurrence of celiac disease in subjects HLADQ2/DQ8 positive: a prospective study. Helicobacter 2018; 23:e12465.

[22] Konturek PC, Karczewska E, DieterichW, Hahn EG, Schuppan D. Increased prevalence of Helicobacter pylori infection in patients with celiac disease. Am J Gastroenterol. 2000; 95:3682-3683.

[23] Uusitalo U, Lee HS, Aronsson CA, Yang J, Virtanen SM, Norris J, Agardh D; Environmental Determinants of the Diabetes in the Young (TEDDY) study group. Gluten consumption during late pregnancy and risk of celiac disease in the offspring: the TEDDY birth cohort. Am J Clin Nutr. 2015; 102:1216-1221.

[24] Emilsson L, Magnus MC, Stordal K. Perinatal risk factors for development of celiac disease in children, based on the prospective Norwegian Mother and Child Cohort Study. Clin Gastroenterol Hepatol. 2015; 13:921-927.

[25] Koletzko S, Lee HS, Beyerlein A, Aronsson CA, Hummel M, Liu E, Simell V, Kurppa K, Lernmark Å, Hagopian W, Rewers M, She JX, Simell O, Toppari J, Ziegler AG, Krischer J, Agardh D; TEDDY Study Group. Cesarean section on the risk of celiac disease in the offspring: the teddy study. J Pediatr Gastroenterol Nutri. 2018; 66:417-424.

[26] Dydensborg Sander S, Hansen AV, Stordal K A. -Andersen MN, Murray JA, Husby S. Mode of delivery is not associated with celiac disease. Clin Epidemiol. 2018; 10:323-332.

[27] Stordal K, Haugen M, Brantsaeter AL, Lundin KE, Stene LC. Association between maternal iron supplementation during pregnancy and risk of celiac disease in children. Clin Gastroenterol Hepatol. 2014; 12:624-31 e1-2.

[28] Yang J, Tamura RN, Aronsson CA, Uusitalo UM, Lernmark Å, Rewers M, Hagopian WA, She JX, Toppari J, Ziegler AG, Akolkar B, Krischer JP, Norris JM, Virtanen SM, Agardh D; Environmental Determinants of Diabetes in The Young study group. Maternal use of dietary supplements during pregnancy is not associated with coeliac disease in the offspring: the environmental determinants of diabetes in the young (TEDDY) study. Br J Nutr. 2017; 117:466-72.

[29] Lebwohl B, Green PH, Murray JA, Ludvigsson JF. Season of birth in a nationwide cohort of coeliac disease patients. Arch Dis Child. 2013; 98:48-51.

[30] Assa A, Waisbourd-Zinman O, Daher S, Shamir R. Birth month as a risk factor for the diagnosis of celiac disease later in life: a population-based study. J Pediatr Gastroenterol Nutr. 2018; 67:367-370.

[31] Ivarsson A, Hernell O, NystromL, Persson LA. Children born in the summer have increased risk for coeliac disease. J Epidemiol Community Health 2003; 57:36-39.

[32] Canova C, Zabeo V, Pitter G, Romor P, Baldovin T, Zanotti R, Simonato L. Association of maternal education, early infections, and antibiotic use with celiac disease: a population-based birth cohort study in northeastern Italy. Am J Epidemiol. 2014; 180: 76-85.

[33] Wijarnpreecha K, Lou S, Panjawatanan P, Cheungpasitporn W, Pungpapong S, Lukens FJ, Ungprasert P. Cigarette smoking and risk of celiac disease: a systematic review and meta-analysis. United European Gastroenterol J. 2018; 6: 1285-1293.

[34] Kondrashova A, Mustalahti K, Kaukinen K, Viskari H, Volodicheva V, Haapala AM, Ilonen J, Knip M, Mäki M, Hyöty H; Epivir Study Group. Lower economic status and inferior hygienic environment may protect against celiac disease. Ann Med. 2008; 40:223-231.

[35] Roy A, Mehra S, Kelly CP, Tariq S, Pallav K, Dennis M, Peer A, Lebwohl B, Green PH, Leffler DA. The association between socioeconomic status and the symptoms at diagnosis of celiac disease: a retrospective cohort study. Therap Adv Gastroenterol. 2016; 9:495-502.

[36] Unalp-Arida A, Ruhl CE, Choung RS, Brantner TL, Murray JA. Lower prevalence of celiac disease and gluten-related disorders in persons living in Southern vs Northern Latitudes of the United States. Gastroenterology 2017; 152:1922-32.e2.

[37] Teresi S, Crapisi M, Vallejo MD, Castellaneta SP, Francavilla R, Iacono G, Ravelli A, Menegazzi P, Louali M, Catassi C. Celiac disease seropositivity in Saharawi children: a followup and family study. J Pediatr Gastroenterol Nutr. 2010; 50:506-509.

[38] Lionetti E, Gatti S, Pulvirenti A, Catassi C. Celiac disease from a global perspective. Best Pract Res Clin Gastroenterol. 2015; 29:365-379.

[39] Mårild K, Tapia G, Haugen M, Dahl SR, Cohen AS, Lundqvist M, Lie BA, Stene LC, Størdal K. Maternal and neonatal vitamin D status, genotype and childhood celiac disease. PLoS ONE. 2017; 12:e0179080.

[40] Kemppainen KM, Vehik K, Lynch KF, Larsson HE, Canepa RJ,

Simell V, Koletzko S, Liu E, Simell OG, Toppari J, Ziegler AG, Rewers MJ, Lernmark Å, Hagopian WA, She JX, Akolkar B, Schatz DA, Atkinson MA, Blaser MJ, Krischer JP, Hyöty H, Agardh D, Triplett EW; Environmental Determinants of Diabetes in the Young (TEDDY) Study Group. Association between early-life antibiotic use and the risk of islet or celiac disease autoimmunity. JAMA Pediatr. 2017; 171:1217-1225.

[41] Lebwohl B, Spechler SJ, Wang TC, Green PH, Ludvigsson JF. Use of proton pump inhibitors and subsequent risk of celiac disease. Dig Liver Dis. 2014; 46:36-40.

[42] Carroccio A, Di Prima L, Noto D, Fayer F, Ambrosiano G, Villanacci V, Lammers K, Lafiandra D, De Ambrogio E, Di Fede G, Iacono G, Pogna N. Searching for wheat plants with low toxicity in celiac disease: between direct toxicity and immunologic activation. Dig Liver Dis. 2011; 43: 34-39.

[43] International Wheat Genome Sequencing Consortium (IWGSC), et al. Shifting the limits in wheat research and breeding using a fully annotated reference genome. Science. 2018; 361: eaar7191.

[44] Pinier M, Verdu EF, Nasser-Eddine M, David CS, Vézina A, Rivard N, Leroux JC. Polymeric binders suppress gliadin-induced toxicity in the intestinal epithelium. Gastroenterology. 2009; 136:288-298.

[45] Pinier M, Fuhrmann G, Galipeau HJ, Rivard N, Murray JA, David CS, Drasarova H, Tuckova L, Leroux JC, Verdu EF. The copolymer P(HEMA-co-SS) binds gluten and reduces immune response in gluten-sensitized mice and human tissues. Gastroenterology. 2012; 142:316-25.e1-12.

[46] McCarville JL, Nisemblat Y, Galipeau HJ, Jury J, Tabakman R, Cohen A, Naftali E, Neiman B, Halbfinger E, Murray JA, Anbazhagan AN, Dudeja PK, Varvak A, Leroux JC, Verdu EF. BL-7010 demonstrates specific binding to gliadin and reduces glutenassociated pathology in a chronic mouse model of gliadin sensitivity. PLoS ONE. 2014; 9:e109972.

[47] Gujral N, Löbenberg R, Suresh M, Sunwoo H. In-vitro and in-vivo binding activity of chicken egg yolk immunoglobulin Y (IgY) against gliadin in food matrix. J Agric Food Chem. 2012; 60:3166-3172.

[48] Sample DA, Sunwoo HH, Huynh HQ, Rylance HL, Robert CL, Xu BW, Kang SH, Gujral N, Dieleman LA. AGY, a novel egg yolk-derived anti-gliadin antibody, is safe for patients with Celiac disease. Dig Dis Sci. 2017; 62:1277-1285.

[49] Paterson BM, Lammers KM, ArrietaMC, Fasano A,Meddings JB. The safety, tolerance, pharmacokinetic and pharmacodynamic effects of single doses of AT-1001 in coeliac disease subjects: a proof of concept study. Aliment Pharmacol Ther. 2007; 26:757-766.

[50] Leffler DA, Kelly CP, Abdallah HZ, Colatrella AM, Harris LA, Leon F, Arterburn LA, Paterson BM, Lan ZH, Murray JA. A randomized, double-blind study of larazotide acetate to prevent the activation of celiac disease during gluten challenge. Am J Gastroenterol. 2012; 107:1554-1562.

[51] Kelly CP, Green PHR, Murray JA, Dimarino A, Colatrella A, Leffler DA, Alexander T, Arsenescu R, Leon F, Jiang JG, Arterburn LA, Paterson BM, Fedorak RN. Larazotide acetate in patients with coeliac disease undergoing a gluten challenge: a randomised

placebo-controlled study. Aliment
Pharmacol Ther. 2013; 37:252-262.

[52] Leffler DA, Kelly CP, Green PHR,
Fedorak RN, DiMarino A, Perrow W,
Rasmussen H, Wang C, Bercik P,
Bachir NM, Murray JA. Larazotide
acetate for persistent symptoms of celiac
disease despite a gluten-free diet: a
randomized controlled trial.
Gastroenterology. 2015; 148:1311-9.e6.

Chapter 2

The Association of HLA-DQ2 with Celiac Disease

Federica Gualandris, Laura Castellani and Anna Falanga

Abstract

DQ2 is a surface receptor of class II MHC exposed on APC immune-competent cells. Its function is to recognize non-self-antigens and present them to CD4+ T-helper lymphocytes, which activate cytokine <21> production and control antibody production and cell response. The activation of T lymphocytes by peptides derived from gluten proteins and the production of antibodies directed against tTG in tissues where it is localized is the basis of the etiopathogenesis of celiac disease (CD). CD is frequently associated with the presence of specific HLA system genes encoding heterodimers DQ2 and DQ8, identifiable by the DQA1*0501/DQB1*0201 or DQA1*0501/DQB1*0202 and DQB1*0302 alleles. DQ2 is also associated with genetic, endocrinological and neurological diseases such as: type 1 diabetes, thyroiditis, pancreatitis and multiple sclerosis. Interactions between DQ2 and T lymphoma have also been demonstrated. The correlation between autoimmune diseases in patients with CD and therefore DQ2 is much more frequent than in healthy subjects.

Keywords: HLA-DQ2, DQ2 isoforms, DQ2 and celiac disease, DQ2 and diseases, T helper lymphocytes

1. Introduction to HLA-DQ2 structure and localization

HLA-DQ2 antigen is a surface receptor of antigen-presenting cells (APC), it is composed of two polypeptide subunits: the α chain (of 32–34 kD) and the β chain (of 29–32 kD) [1]. Each one presents a peptide-binding domain, an Ig-like domain, and a transmembrane region with a cytoplasmic tail (**Figure 1**). These structures are bind by non-covalent association leadings. Unlike Major Histocompatibility Complex (MHC) class I molecules, both polypeptide chains are encoded by genes in the HLA-DQ regions strictly located on chromosome 6 (**Figure 2**). The pocket for the bond with the peptide is constituted for half by one chain and half by the other; each one contributes with an α-helix and 4 filaments of the β sheet.

In the extracellular portion, each chain has an Ig domain (α2 and β2) of which, β2 contains the binding site for lymphocyte helper CD4+. In HLA-DQ2 both the α-chains and the β-chains are polymorphic, as a result, unique DQ molecules can be formed, with α- and β-chains encoded on the same chromosome (encoded in cis) or on opposite chromosomes (encoded in trans). However, evidence suggests that not every α- and β-chain pairing will form a stable heterodimer. It is generally considered that alleles of DQα- and DQβ-chains pair up predominantly in cis rather than in trans. However, the occurrence of trans-encoded HLA class II molecules is well

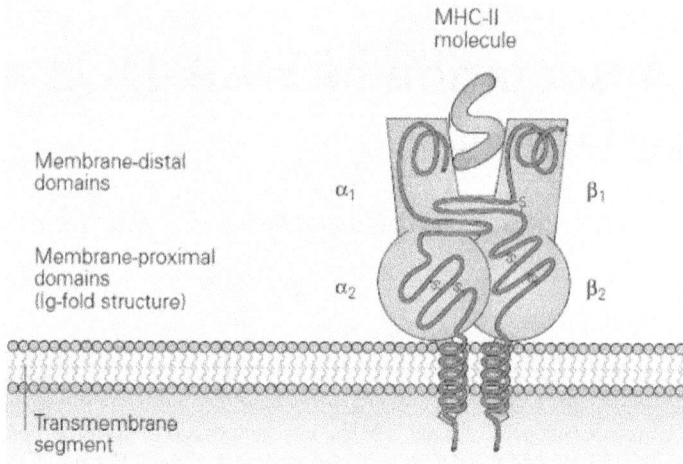

Figure 1.
Label: The structure of the MHC-II molecule [2].

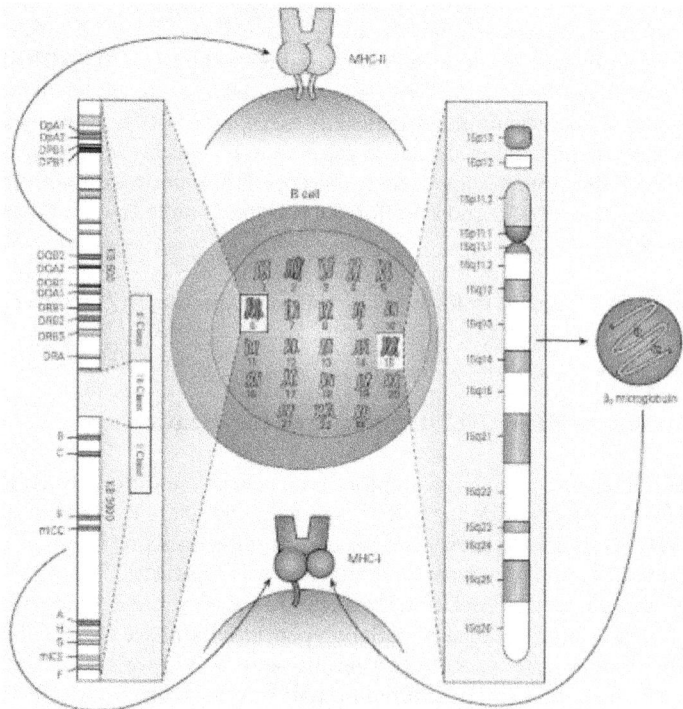

Figure 2.
Label: Chromosomal origin of HLA class I and class II [3].

documented in the literature, such as in the case of type 1 diabetes (T1D), where the trans encoded HLA molecules may play a role in pathogenesis [4].

Each MHC molecule has only one antigen pocket that can bind one peptide at once, but different peptides at different times. Peptides that can bind to MHC-II molecules reach 30 or more, while class I MHC molecules can accommodate peptides with 8–11 amino acids. The peptide–MHC binding is created during its assembly and is used to stabilize the complex to allow its expression on the cell surface and for this reason, the dissociation rate is very slow. This naturally provides a very long half-life that allows T lymphocytes to meet the antigen. Between MHC and peptide, a non-covalent connection is formed among the residues in the pocket. Once the binding has occurred, the peptide and the water molecules that solubilize it fill the pocket, making contact with the walls and the floor that make it up.

T cells activated by class II molecules are CD4+ helper cells that: activate cytokine production, control antibody synthesis, and regulate cellular response. DQ is also involved in the common recognition of auto-antigens; the presentation of these antigens to the immune system provides tolerance at a young age. When this tolerance is lost DQ can be involved in autoimmune diseases such as celiac disease (CD), type 1 diabetes, and many others as we will see more details afterward [5].

2. HLA-DQ2 isoforms

As mentioned before, there are many potential DQ isoforms, as a result of the combination of cis- and trans haplotypes and those with cis-pairing are more common. Typically individuals can produce 4 isoforms, but only HLA-DQ2.5 and HLA-DQ2.2 tend to be predominantly represented.

HLA-DQ2.5 is composed of the allele HLA-DQA1*0501 (or DQA1*0505) encoding the alpha chain and the allele HLA-DQB1*0201 (or DQB1*0202) encoding the beta chain. HLA-DQ2.2 consists of the HLA-DQA1*02 alpha chain allele and the HLA-DQB1*0202 beta chain allele [6].

Very important concerning isoforms is that different subunit matches can cause the binding of different foreign or self-antigens. Generally, MHC molecules have slots at the pocket level that can interact with specific amino acids or be complementary to certain amino acid side chains. The importance of polymorphism is detected here: only the ability of MHC to bind specifically to a peptide permits it to be recognized by lymphocytes and to trigger the immune response to it.

The molecule HLA-DQ2 has a peculiar ligation system with three binding sites, preferably for negatively charged residues and different peptide-binding motifs. The binding motifs associated with HLA-DQ2 consist of truncated variants of eight different peptides with a length of 9–19 amino acids.

Data from the pooled sequencing and the biochemical binding analyses of synthetic variants of a ligand indicate that the side chains of amino acid residues at relative position P1 (bulky hydrophobic), P4 (negatively charged or aliphatic), P6 (Pro or negatively charged), P7 (negatively charged) and P9 (bulky hydrophobic) are important for binding of peptides to DQ2 (**Figure 3**).

Computer modeling of the DQ2 with variants of the ligand in the groove suggests that peptides bind to DQ2 through the primary anchors P1, P7, and P9 and making additional advantageous interactions using the P4 and P6 positions [8].

2.1 HLA-DQ2.5

DQ2.5 refers to both a protein isoform and a genetic haplotype. DQ2.5 isoform or heterodimer is shorthand for the cell surface receptor HLA-DQ α5β2 (**Figure 4**).

DQ2.5 and the linked DR3 are associated with probably the greatest frequency of autoimmune occurrence relative to any other haplotypes. A genome-wide survey of markers linked to celiac disease, reveals that the highest linkage is for a marker within the DQA1*0501 allele of the DQ2.5 haplotype. The association of DQB1*0201 is almost as high. Greatly elevating risk is the ability of the DQ2.5 haplotype encoded isoforms to increase abundance on the cell surface in DQ2.5 double

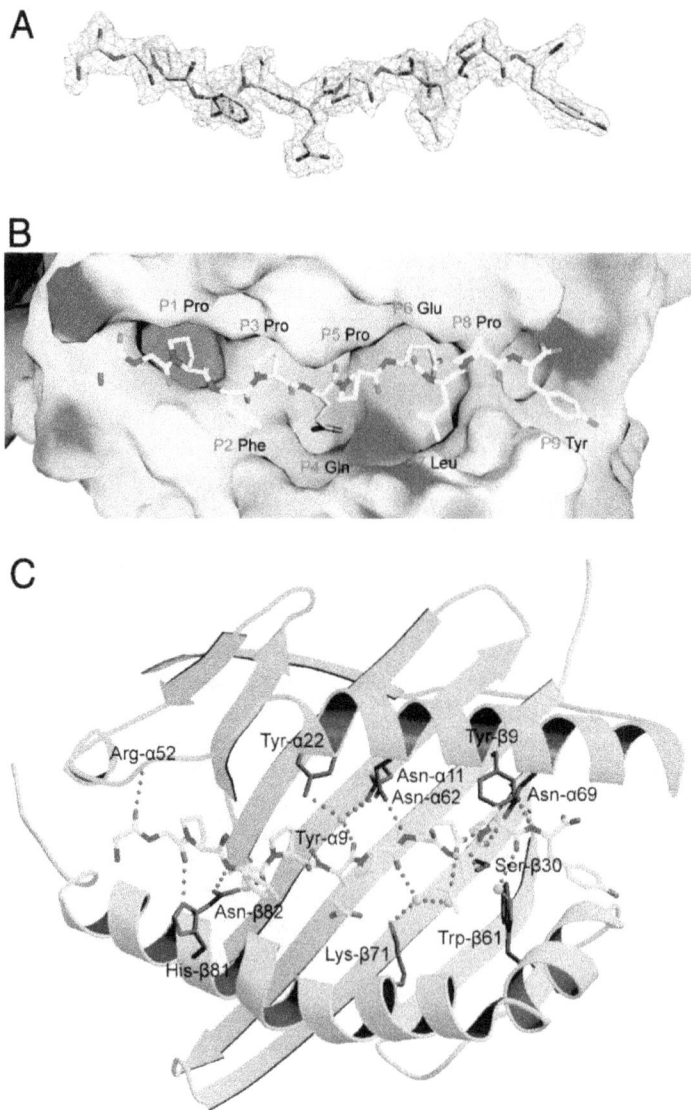

Figure 3.
Label: Analysis of the HLA-DQ2 protein: (A) the 3D structure; (B) the binding sites; (C) the amino acids residues and the α helix and the β sheet domains [7].

homozygote. While the frequency of DQ2.5 haplotype is only 4 times higher than the general population, the number of DQ2.5 homozygotes is 10 to 20 times higher than the general population. Of the approximately 90% of celiacs that bear the DQ2.5 isoform, only 4% produce DQ2.5trans and differs slightly, one amino acid, from DQ2.5cis.

Multiple copies of the DQ2.5 haplotype do not cause apparent increases of severity in celiac disease, but the 25% of celiac patients homozygous DQ2 (DQ2.5/DQ2) tend to show increases risk of life-threatening complications and more severe histological findings. The HLA-DQ2.5 molecule preferentially binds peptides with negatively charged amino acids at anchor positions [10, 11]. Whereas gluten peptides contain few negative charges, these charges can be introduced by

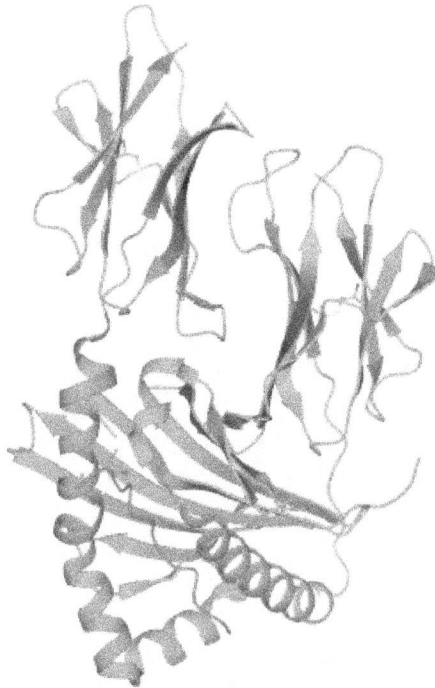

Figure 4.
Label: The crystal structure of HLA-DQ2.5-CLIP1 [9].

the enzyme tissue transglutaminase (tTG) that selectively deamidates glutamine residues in gluten peptides [12–14]. DQ2.5cis is the major factor in adaptive immunity by frequency and efficiency in alpha-gliadin presentation and its responses can be differentiated from other DQ isoforms. Specifically, this DQ2 heterodimer is responsible for presenting the α2-gliadin that most effectively stimulates pathogenic T-cells.

As mentioned before, the DQ2.5 haplotype is linked to DR3, which is not linked to DQ2.2. Using either serotyping or genotyping DQ2.5 can be distinguished from DQ2.2 or DQ2.3 [5].

2.2 HLA-DQ2.2

HLA-DQ2.2 is shorthand for the DQ α2β2 heterodimeric isoform (**Figure 5**). DQ2.2 homozygotes represent about 1.1% of the celiac population. While HLA-DQ2.5 is strongly associated with the disease, HLA-DQ2.2 is not [5].

Whereas the molecular surfaces of the antigen-binding clefts of HLA-DQ2.5 and HLA-DQ2.2 are very similar, there are important differences in the nature of the peptides presented. These peculiarities in peptide motif binding cause differences in responding to T cell repertoires and in the disease penetrance [16].

DQ2.2 individuals can mount an antigluten response but bear a lower risk of celiac disease. The reason is fewer gluten peptides would bind stably to this HLA molecule. The results give insight into processes important for the establishment of T-cell responses to antigen in HLA-associated diseases. Patients with celiac disease with DQ2.2 have gluten-reactive T cells in their small intestine [17].

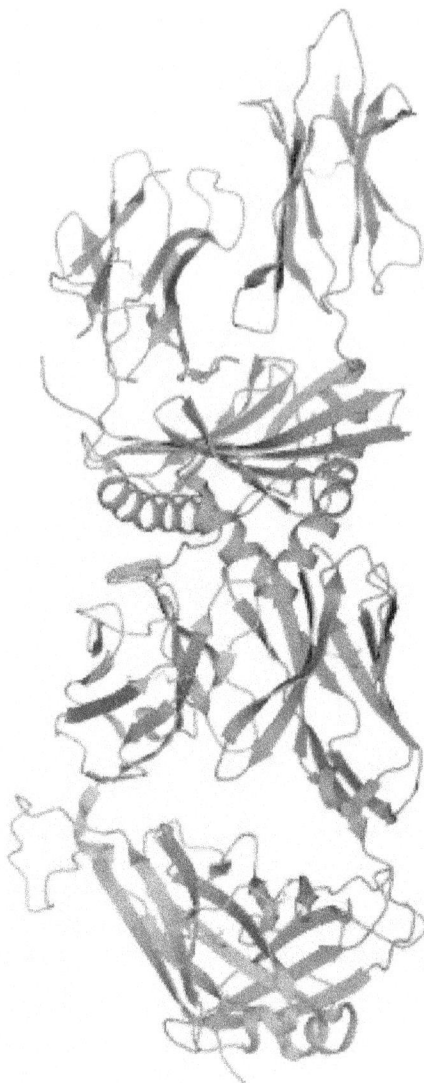

Figure 5.
Label: The crystal structure of HLA-DQ2.2 [15].

2.3 HLA-DQ2.3

DQ2.3 is the shorthand for the heterodimeric DQ α3β2 isoform and is encoded by the DQA1*03:DQB1*02 haplotype (**Figure 6**). The receptor coded for the haplotype is a DQ2.3cis isoform, which is genetically linked to DR7 [5]. The gluten epitope, which is the only known HLA-DQ2.3-restricted epitope, is preferentially recognized in the context of the DQ2.3 molecule by the T-cell clones of a DQ8/DQ2.5 heterozygous celiac patient.

The DQ2.3 molecule combines the peptide binding signatures of the DQ2.5 and DQ8 molecules. This results in a binding motif with a preference for negatively charged anchor residues at both the P1 and the P4 positions. In this way, some epitopes can be presented even more effectively in the context of the trans-encoded

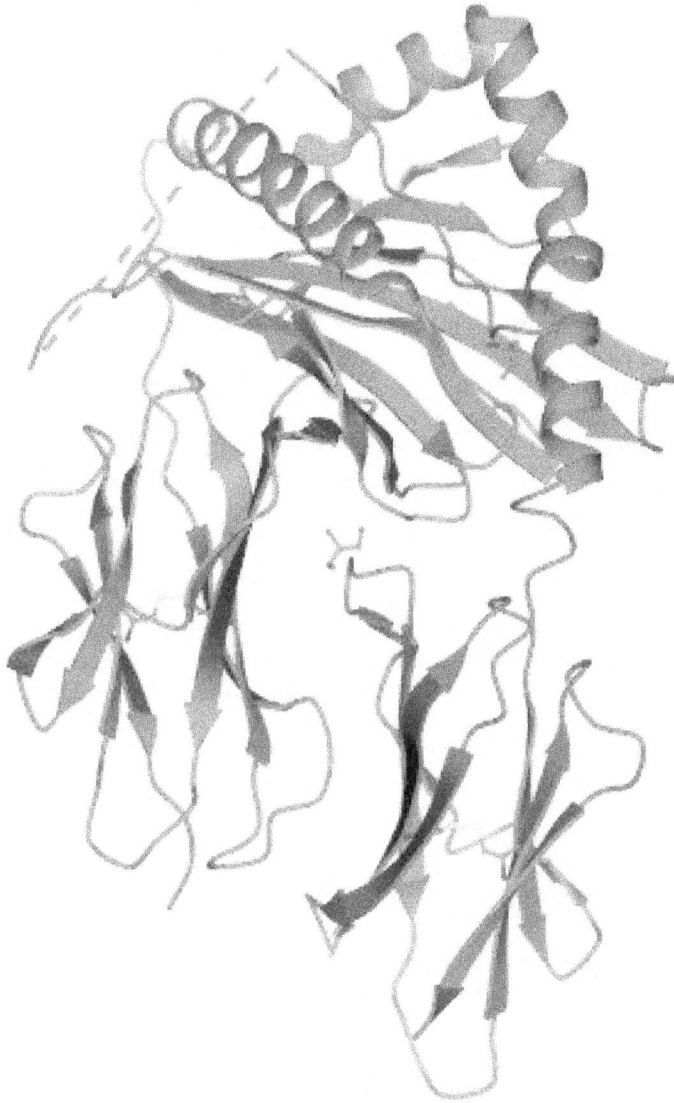

Figure 6.
Label: The crystal structure of HLA-DQ2.3 [18].

DQ2.3 molecule. This has relevance for understanding how the trans-encoded DQ2.3 molecule is predisposing to type 1 diabetes [4].

The analysis of the structure of DQ2.3 together with all other available DQ crystals shows that the P1 pocket in DQ2.3 is significantly different from that of DQ2.5 due to the polymorphic MHC residues found in this region. Additionally, DQ2.3 presents a gluten epitope to T-cells much more efficiently than DQ2.5 [4].

3. Other isoforms

DQ2 beta chains can combine with trans chains to other alpha chains. However, there is no preference in cis isoforms for DQ2 alpha chains, 4, 7, 8, or 9 bindings to DQ1 alpha chains (DQA1*01). The DQA1*03, *05 chains process nearly identical alpha chains. The *04 chain can potentially combine with DQ2 to form DQ2.4. There is the possibility of DQ2.6 resulting from coupling with DQA1*0601 [5].

4. HLA-DQ2 and celiac disease

Celiac disease is a genetically determined immune-mediated disorder in which individuals carrying HLA DQ2 and/or DQ8 haplotypes develop an immuno-logic response to gluten ingestion that leads to a wide range of clinical signs and symptoms.

The Humoral nature, the hereditary and the polygenic CD have great influence in triggering the disease. The assessment of HLA-DQ2/DQ8 is relevant from a diagnostic aspect to detect celiac disease; in fact, about 95% of patients with CD present the HLA-DQ2 genotype [19].

In celiac patient inflammatory T cell responses to HLA-DQ2-bound gluten peptides are thought to cause disease. Gluten-reactive T cells can be isolated from small intestinal biopsies of celiac patients. T cells derived from the lesion mainly recognize gluten deamidate peptides. There are several distinct T cell epitopes within gluten. DQ2 and DQ8 bind the epitopes so that the glutamic acid residues created by deamidification are placed in compartments that have a preference for negatively charged side chains. Evidence indicates that in vivo deamidation is mediated by the enzyme tissue transglutaminase (tTG) that can also cross-link glutamine residues of peptides with lysine residues in other proteins, including tTG itself. This can lead to the formation of gluten-tTG complexes. These complexes may allow gluten-reactive T-cells to provide aid to tTG-specific B-cells through an intramolecular aid mechanism, thus explaining the presence of gluten-dependent tTG autoantibodies which is a characteristic feature of active CDs.

5. HLA-DQ2 and celiac disease class risk

Ideally, all patients with CD carry alleles encoding for the DQ2 and/or DQ8 molecules or at least one chain of the DQ2 heterodimer. The presence of CD in the absence of these DQ risk factors is extremely rare. The presence of these molecules does not accurately predict that CD will develop, as they are present in 25–50% of the general population, although the fact that the vast majority of these individuals will never develop the disease. About 90% of individuals with CD carry HLA-DQ2.5, while individuals with CD who do not express these haplotype usually express either HLA-DQ2.2 or HLA-DQ8; very few coding for HLA DQ7.5 (DQA1*05:05–DQB1*03:01), DQ2.3 or DQ8.5 (DQA1*05–DQB1*03:02).

Differences in CD risk between haplotypes are related to gluten peptide binding and subsequent T-cell response. The effect of gene dose is related to the level of peptide binding to homozygous and heterozygous HLA-DQ2 and its subsequent presentation to T cells. Individuals homozygous for DQ2.5 and DQ8 have an increased risk of the disease. Gluten presentation by HLA-DQ2 homozygous was superior to HLA-DQ2/non-DQ2 in terms of T cell proliferation and cytokine secretion (**Figure** 7).

HLA-DQ2.5 predisposes to celiac disease respect to DQ2.2, because the first one presents a large repertoire of gluten peptides, whereas the second one presents only a subset of these. HLA-DQ2.2 does not predispose to CD unless it is expressed in combination with HLA-DQ2.5. Gluten presentation by HLA-DQ2.5/2.2 induces intermediate T-cell stimulation. However, individuals homozygous for HLA-DQ2.5

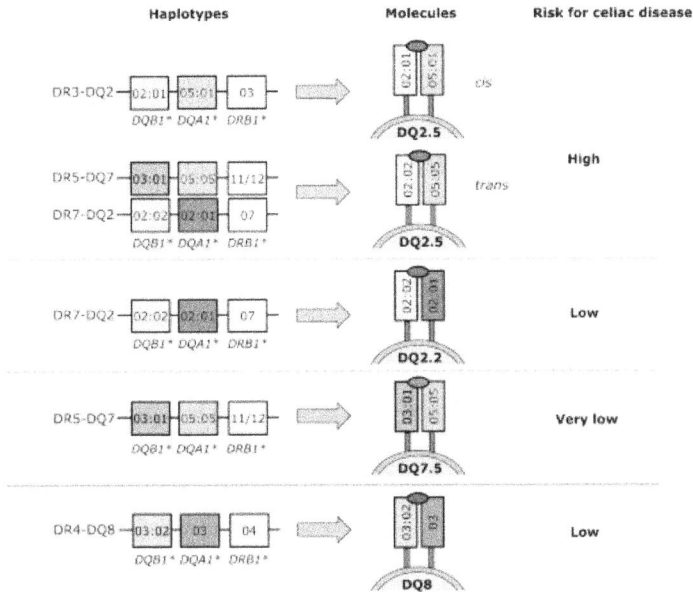

Figure 7.
Label: Haplotypes and different class risk for celiac disease [20].

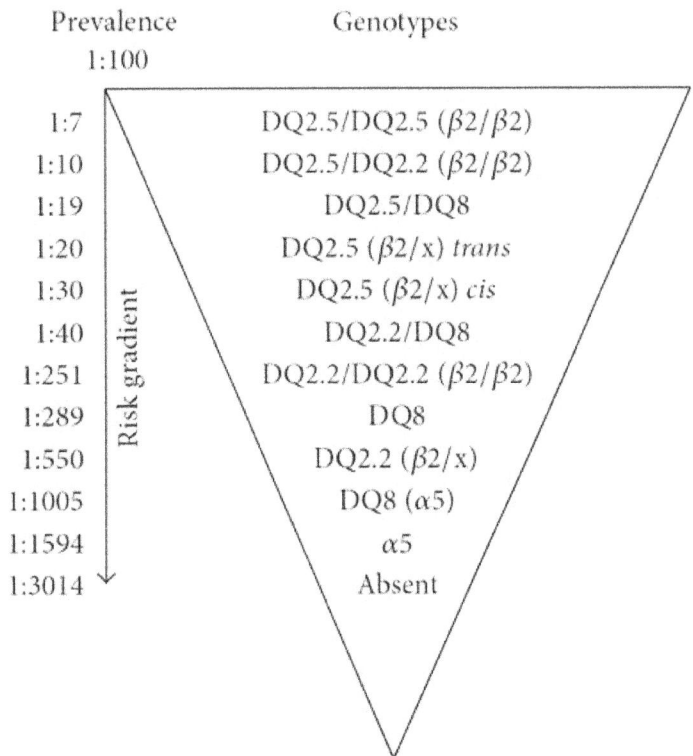

Figure 8.
Label: Genotypes and celiac disease prevalence [21].

or heterozygous HLA-DQ2.2/2.5 have the highest risk of developing CD. In HLA-DQ2.5/2.2 heterozygous individuals have properties identical with HLA-DQ2.5 dimers. In contrast, HLA-DQ2.5/non-DQ2.2 heterozygous individuals have an only slightly increased risk (**Figure 8**).

Considering even more in detail, it has been demonstrated that differences in conferred risk associated with CD are the result of the polymorphism in the α chain between HLA-DQ2.5 and HLA-DQ2.2.

HLA-DQ2.2 is virtually identical to the peptide-binding properties of HLA-DQ2.5. Both are highly homologous except for a single polymorphic residue (HLA-DQ2.5-Tyr22α and HLA-DQ2.2-Phe22α). The role of the Phe22α variant in HLA-DQ2.2 is to influence peptide binding preferences and to decide how DQ2.2 TCRs engage the DQ2.2-gluten complex.

Crystal structure studies revealed a docking strategy, where the TCR HLA-DQ2.5 gliadin epitopes complexes were notably distinct from the HLA-DQ2.2-glut TCR complex [22].

HLA-DQ2.5 and HLA-DQ2.2 binds and presents gluten peptides with glutamate residues at anchor positions P4, P6, or P7). Three HLA-DQ2.2 epitopes (DQ2.2-glut-L1, DQ2.2-glia-α1, and DQ2.2-glia-α2) have sequences similar to HLADQ2.5 binding peptides, with the exception that they all carry serine at P3. As seen for HLA-DQ2.5 epitopes, the HLA-DQ2.2 ones display a hierarchy with DQ2.2-glut-L1 being the epitopes recognized by most T cells [23].

6. HLA-DQ2 and interaction with HLA-DM

HLA-DQ2 is influenced by interaction with Ag presentation cofactors, invariant chain (Ii), HLA-DM (DM), a peptide exchange catalyst for MHC class II (**Figure 9**).

DM can enhance or suppress the presentation of specific MHCII peptide complexes. In general, MHCII–peptide complexes with lower intrinsic stability are DM susceptible, but not all high-stability complexes are DM resistant. HLA-DQ2 is relatively resistant to DM because DQ2 has a natural deletion in the region involved in the interaction with DM, compared with most other alleles.

The role of DQ2/DM concerns interaction in the DQ2-restricted gliadin epitopes, relevant to celiac disease, or DQ2-restricted viral epitopes, relevant to host defense. DM activity has different consequences on DQ2 presentation of epitopes to T cell clones, with suppression of gliadin presentation and enhancement of viral peptide presentation. These results imply key differences in DQ2 Ag presentation pathways.

DM-resistant feature of DQ2 likely contributes to the escape of gliadin peptides from extensive DM editing. Also, DQ2 has the special ability to stably bind proline-rich gliadin peptides that use TG2-deamidated residues as DQ2-binding anchors.

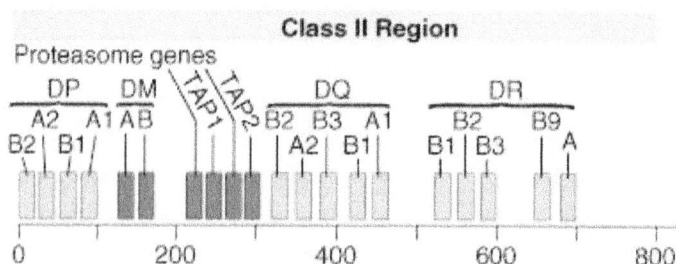

Figure 9.
Label: Localization of HLA-DM on the MHC class II region [24].

Together, these unique features of DQ2 may allow gliadin presentation to disease-driving CD4$^+$ T cells and contribute to the uniquely selective DQ2 presentation of DM-sensitive gliadin epitopes.

In contrast, the presentation of DM-resistant epitopes that form more-stable complexes with DQ2 likely relies less on the above mechanisms, as DM editing positively affects the presentation of these epitopes. The elevation of DM expression in peripheral APC (particularly during infection) may benefit self-tolerance by attenuating the presentation of DM-sensitive epitopes while boosting the presentation of DM-resistant pathogen-derived epitopes and aiding in host defense [25].

7. HLA-DQ2 refractory celiac disease (RCD) and enteropathy-associated T-cell lymphoma (EATL)

Refractory celiac disease (RCD) is defined by persistent mal-absorptive symptoms and villous atrophy despite strict adherence to a GFD for at least 6–12 months in the absence of other causes of non-responsive treated celiac disease.

The pathology can be classified as type 1 (normal intraepithelial lymphocyte phenotype), or type 2 (defined by the presence of abnormal [clonal] intraepithelial lymphocyte phenotype). RCD 1 usually improves after treatment with a combination of aggressive nutritional support, adherence to GFD, and alternative pharmacologic therapies. By contrast, clinical response to alternative therapies in RCD 2 is less certain and the prognosis is poor. Severe complications such as ulcerative jejunity and Enteropathy T-cell lymphoma (ETL) may occur in a subgroup of patients with RCD [26].

ETL is a T-cell non-Hodgkin lymphoma arising in the gastrointestinal tract that shows a differentiation of tumor cells toward the phenotype of intestinal intraepithelial T cells. The clinical course of ETL is highly aggressive, with most patients dying from the disease within months of diagnosis. Enteropathy T-cell lymphoma comprises two morphologically, clinically, and genetically distinct lymphoma entities: the ETL type 1 and 2.

ETL arises in individuals with the DQA1*0501, DQB1*02 CD-predisposing genotype. The HLA typing found in these patients revealed that more than 95% have an HLA-DQ2/-DQ8 genotype [27]. Comparing studies of HLA-DQB1 genotyping in celiac disease and ETL have detected that the overall HLA-DQB1 genotype pattern observed in type 1 ETL closely resembled those for ETL, whereas those of type 2 ETL are not significantly different from that of normal Caucasian controls.

ETL1 patients show significantly more frequent expression of HLA-DQB1*02 than the type 2 ones [28]. Lymphoma type 1 may arise and be pathogenetically linked to refractory celiac disease by a stepwise acquisition of genetic alterations. Contrary given the genetic alterations and HLA-DQB1 genotype patterns, celiac disease may not be causal to type 2 ETL. At least 47% of patients with type 2 ETL are very likely to never have had celiac disease [29].

The highly significant correlation between HLA-DQ2 homozygosity and the development of RCD II and ETL, suggests that the strength of the gluten-specific T-cell response in the laminapropria directly or indirectly influences the likelihood of RCD II and lymphoma development. As already mentioned in the chapter, also in this case, the higher T-cell proliferation and cytokine secretion induced by HLA-DQ2 homozygous APC, than HLA-DQ2 heterozygous APC, may explain the strongly increased risk for disease development in HLA-DQ2/DQ2 individuals [30]. This would indicate that adherence to a gluten-free diet is particularly important for CD patients who are HLA-DQ2 homozygous.

These observations suggest that specific tests, such as those for lymphocyte typing for T cells, should be indicated in all patients with CD who are not responding to a gluten-free diet. The availability of a simple and reliable immune histochemical method can make the distinction between CD and RCD feasible. HLA-DQ typing is doable and it may be an efficient test to recognize individuals at risk for these conditions with a poor prognosis, particularly now that some evidence has been given to support the hypothesis that autologous hematopoietic stem-cell transplantation can alter disease progression in severe [29].

8. HLA-DQ2 and liver/gastrointestinal (GI) disease

Liver and gastrointestinal diseases have many etiologies that are poorly understood. Whether due to genetic abnormalities, psychological factors, or other environmental variables, functional disorders can be complex and difficult cases to resolve. A strongest evidence of an association with *DQ2/8* was found in patients with functional upper GI disorders [31]. There are several reasons why it may be prudent to study DQ2/8 alleles in GI disease outside of celiac disease in fact, evidence suggests that celiac disease may alter the risk of developing irritable bowel syndrome (IBS), inflammatory bowel disease (IBD), eosinophilic esophagitis, or certain liver diseases. Several studies have directly compared the prevalence of the DQ2/8 haplotype in GI disease. These haplotypes may play a role in liver/digestive disease through pathological mechanisms different from those of celiac disease. DQ2/8 contains myriad genes involved in inflammatory processes, such as tumor necrosis factor-α, causal mechanisms between these genes, and GI disease may exist.

Known immunological associations between IBD and DR7, which is linked to both DQ2 and DQ8 haplotype have been established. The relation between DQ2/8 and IBD/IBS was analyzed in particular in two studies from an Italian and a Danish group and both demonstrated that the proportion of IBS was lower among HLA DQ2/8 positive individuals. However the Italian group also found that IBD and liver diseases were more prevalent among HLADQ2/8 subjects, but it is not confirmed in the Danish study. Prior prevalence data though suggest that IBD, particularly Crohn's disease, is lower in individuals with the DQ2/8 linked celiac disease.

IBS has also been linked to HLA DQ2/8 haplotypes and intestinal transit rates [31]. Approximately 46% of patients with diarrhea-predominant IBS (IBS-D) have accelerated colonic transit. Some patients with IBS report an association of symptoms with specific foods, suggesting a role for food hypersensitivity. One such food is gluten in the absence of overt celiac disease. The spectrum of gluten sensitivity ranges from minimal histological changes such as increased intraepithelial lymphocytes without villous atrophy, increased immunoglobulin A (IgA) deposits in intestinal villi, gluten-sensitive diarrhea, and immunological mucosal response to gluten exclusion in patients with celiac disease. Typically, one or more of these findings are seen in individuals who are positive for HLA-DQ2 or HLA-DQ8. Wahnschaffe et al. demonstrated that, among patients with IBS-D, response of diarrhea to a gluten-free diet was influenced by HLA-DQ2 positivity and the presence of IgG tissue transglutaminase (TTG) antibody in duodenal aspirates. Symptom response to gluten withdrawal occurred in 62% of patients positive for both HLA-DQ2 and IgG-TTG; in contrast, only 12% of patients negative for HLA-DQ2 and TTG-IgG responded; suggesting that symptom generation in this subset of patients is immune-mediated. Is demonstrated that patients with IBS-D, positive for either HLA-DQ8 or both HLA-DQ2/DQ8 genotypes that are associated with gluten sensitivity, have an accelerated colonic transit time [32].

The HLA DQ2 in association with HLA-DR3 is also associated with another GI disease; in fact, this combination is linked with a more rapid progression of primary sclerosing cholangitis (PSC) [33].

9. HLA-DQ2 and diabetes

Type 1 diabetes (T1D) is an autoimmune disease attacking pancreatic Langerhans islets. The islets are composed of several types of cells: α, β, δ, ε, and pancreatic polypeptide (PP). Each type plays a different role in the secretory function of the pancreas and, among others, α and β cells produce glucagon and insulin, respectively. The interplay between these two compounds provides proper glucose level administration in blood.

It has been already shown that auto aggression in T1D starts in mutations in the MHC system. HLA-DQ molecules have the role to bind and present beta-cell autoantigen derived peptides in T1D. The combinations of DR4-DQ8 and DR3-DQ2 antigens occur in 90% of people with diabetes. However, the homozygous state for an allele does not further increase the risk. Indeed it is well established that individuals heterozygous for HLA-DQ2 and HLA-DQ8 have almost 5 fold higher risk than homozygous to development of T1D [1, 13, 14]. This has been linked to the formation of trans dimers between the HLA-DQ2 α chain and the HLA-DQ8 β chain (HLA-DQ8 trans) [19, 22, 26, 34]. In particular, the HLA DQ8 trans heterodimer confers the highest risk for the development of T1D. This indicates that such HLA-DQ trans dimers can bind and present a unique autoantigen derived peptide that leads to beta-cell destruction in the pancreas and the development of T1D [35].

Juvenile diabetes has a high association with DQ2.5. A combination of DQ2.5 and DQ8 significantly increases the risk of type 1 onset of adult diabetes, while the presence of DQ2 with DR3 reduces the age of onset and severity of the autoimmune disease.

The formation of trans encoded molecules DQ8.5 (DQA1*05:01/DQB1*03:02) and DQ2.3 (DQA1*03:01/DQB1*02:01), which could present one or a few specific diabetogenic epitopes to CD4+ T-cells, possibly inducing an immune response that leads to the destruction of insulin-producing pancreatic β islet cells [12]. A strong argument for the involvement of the DQ2.3 heterodimer in type 1 diabetes comes from trans racial gene mapping studies that have found that this heterodimer, which is typically found in the trans configuration among Caucasian subjects, exists and is over-represented in the cis configuration among type 1 diabetes patients of African origin [16, 17]. The increased diabetes risk of the African DQ2.3 (DQA1*03:01/DQB1*02) carrying DR7 haplotype is contrasted by a protecting effect of the DQ2.2 (DQA1*03:01/DQB1*02) carrying DR7 haplotype of European origin [17].

Patients with homozygous type 1 DQ2 diabetes have a marked prevalence of IgA anti-transglutaminase autoantibodies. The great excess of positive transglutaminase autoantibodies among homozygous DQ2 diabetics is related to both the presence of DQ2 and its addition to all genetic or environmental factors associated with type 1 diabetes. These additional factors may be related to abnormalities in mucosal immunity that increases the risk of both type 1 diabetes and celiac disease.

Type 1 diabetes is an autoimmune disease attacking pancreatic Langerhan's islet. The islet is composed of several types of cells: α, β, δ, ε, and pancreatic polypeptide (PP). Each type plays a different role in the secretory function of the pancreas and, among others, α and β cells produce glucagon ad insulin, respectively [36]. Interplay between these two compounds provides proper glucose level administration in blood.

It has been already shown that auto aggression in T1D starts in mutation in the MHC system. HLA-DQ molecules have the role to bind and present beta cell auto-antigens derived peptides in T1D. The combinations of DR4-DQ8 and DR3-DQ2 antigens occur in 90% of people with diabetes. However, the homozygous state for an allele does not further increase the risk. It is well established that individuals het-erozygous for HLA-DQ2 and HLA-DQ8 have an almost 5 fold higher risk than those who are homozygous for either of the DQ variants for the development of T1D, and this has been linked to the formation of trans dimers between the HLA-DQ2 α chain and the HLA-DQ8 β chain (HLA-DQ8 trans). This indicates that such HLA-DQ trans dimers can bind and present a unique auto antigen-derived peptide that leads to beta-cell destruction in the pancreas and the development of T1D. In particular, HLA DQ8 trans heterodimer confers the highest risk for the development of T1D.

Indeed diabetes has a high association with DQ2.5. A combination of DQ 2.5 and DQ8 significantly increases the risk of type 1 onset of adult diabetes, while the presence of DQ2 with DR3 reduces the age of onset and severity of the autoimmune disease.

The formation of trans encoded molecules DQ8.5 (DQA1*05:01/ DQB1*03:02) and DQ2.3 (DQA1*03:01/DQB1*02:01), which could present one or a few specific diabetogenic epitopes to CD4+ T cells, possibly inducing an immune response that leads to the destruction of insulin-producing pancreatic β islet cells. Moreover, a strong argument for the involvement of DQ2.3 heterodimer in type 1 diabetes comes from transracial gene mapping studies that have found that this heterodimer, which is typically found in the trans-configuration among Caucasian subject, exists and is over-represented in the cis configuration among type 1 diabetes patients of African origin. The increased diabetes risk of the Africans DQ2.3 carrying DR7 haplotype is contrasted by a protecting effect of the DQ2.2 carrying DR7 haplotype of European origin, speaking to the functional importance of α chain in the DQ2.3 molecule.

Patients with homozygous type 1 DQ2 diabetes have a marked prevalence of IgA anti-transglutaminase autoantibodies. The great excess of positive transglutaminase autoantibodies among homozygous DQ2 diabetics is related to both the presence of DQ2 and its addition to all genetic or environmental factors associated with type 1 diabetes. These additional factors may be related to abnormalities in mucosal immunity that increases the risk of both type 1 diabetes and celiac disease. In T1D the risk associates with the HLA-DQ2/8 heterozygous haplotype was found to be increased compared with homozygous HLA-DQ2 or HLA-DQ8 individuals, suggest-ing an epistatic or synergic effect [37].

10. HLA-DQ2 and thyroid disease

The term autoimmune thyroid disease (AITDs) encompasses several different entities characterized by varying degrees of thyroid dysfunction and the presence of serum auto-antibodies against thyroid tissue-specific components, such as thyroglobulin (TG) and thyroid peroxidase (TPO) [34].

Hashimoto's thyroiditis (HT) and Graves' disease (GD) are AITDs with differ-ent physiopathology, being traditionally regarded as two different disease entities. More recent views, in contrast, have considered the hypothesis that there might be a continuum between HT and GD.

Genes of, or closely associated with, the HLA complex are assumed to contribute to the genetic predisposition to AITDs. Genetics plays a prominent role in both the determination of thyroid hormone and thyrotropin (TSH) concentrations and susceptibility to autoimmune thyroid disease. Heritability studies have suggested that up to 67% of circulating thyroid hormone and TSH concentrations are genetically determined, suggesting a genetic basis for narrow intra-individual variation in levels [34]. Until today the mechanisms leading to thyroid autoimmunity are largely unknown.

In 30%–40% of healthy individuals, DQ2, and DQ8 are associated with diseases such as Hashimoto's Thyroiditis. In patients with a CD instead, autoimmune thyroid disease was observed in 14% and 30.3% in adults, while thyroid abnormalities were described in 37.6% and 41.1% in pediatric age.

Noteworthy was the presence of high titers of serum TPO antibodies [11] and serum TG antibodies [12] in the celiac pediatric patients without a gluten-free diet (GFD), these values were reported to return to normal after 2 or 3 years on a GFD. This finding suggests that these antibodies are gluten dependent.

Furthermore has been analyzed the association between Hashimoto's thyroiditis and celiac disease in the Dutch population and it has been demonstrated that HLA DQ2.5 was associated with higher TSH levels. This correlation is not been found for the other thyroid markers (TPO, FT4). A reason could be that TSH is a more sensitive marker for hypothyroidism, as well as the fact that TSH is a quantitative parameter measured in all participants of that study, giving more power to detect differences.

More than doubled GD rates are correlated to the genetic association to the DR3-DQ2 haplotype [38]. A study of Asian Indian patients with Graves' disease revealed a significant increase in the frequency of HLA-DQW2 as compared to the control population [37]. HLA-DQA1*0501 was also shown to be associated with GD in a Caucasian family study [37] but, the primary susceptibility allele in GD is indeed HLA-DR3 [37]. Further analyses have shown that these variants are almost always inherited together in Caucasian populations, so they act as a single genetic factor. These haplotypes are among the crucial genetic factors of celiac disease in European descendants, confirming a strong connection between gluten intolerance and autoimmune thyroid conditions. This theory is confirmed by studies on a large UK Caucasian case–control population, which have shown that the contribution of the HLA class II region to the genetic susceptibility of Graves' disease is due to the haplotype DRB1*0304-DQB1*02-DQA1*0501, with no independent association of any individual allele. However, as a result of strong linkage disequilibrium within the MHC region, it is difficult to assess which loci are acting as primary etiological determinants. The same HLA haplotype is associated with the large multifunctional proteasome 2 loci (LMP-2). The LMP molecules are overexpressed in thyrocytes, the target cells of Graves' disease and the LMP genes are found within the MHC class II region. The LMP genes may therefore play a role in susceptibility to Graves' disease [39].

11. HLA-DQ2 and dermatitis herpetiformis

Dermatitis herpetiformis (DH) is a chronic, pruritic, papulovesicular skin disease of unknown origin. The characteristic rash is symmetrically distributed over the extensor surfaces and buttocks and, also, most patients with DH have asymptomatic gluten-sensitive Enteropathy [40].

All patients with DH had typical clinical and histologic features, as well as granular deposits of IgA at the dermal-epidermal junction. The gastrointestinal lesions are essentially identical to those seen in patients with ordinary CD, although less severe and more patchy. A pathophysiologic link between CD and DH has been suggested by the observation that the skin lesions of DH as well as the abnormalities of the jejunal mucosa regress on a gluten-free diet.

DH is associated with a markedly increased frequency of the HLA class II antigens DR3 and DQ2. The primary HLA association is HLA-DQ2 (expressed in 100% of DH patients), whereas the HLA-DR3 is code in 95% of cases [41]. HLA-DQ8 may therefore be a second HLA susceptibility molecule in DH; all the DH patients carrying DQ2 plus a DR4 haplotype also carried DQ8.

An increased frequency of DR3, DQ2 homozygosity, and a slightly increased frequency of DR3, DQ2 heterozygosity were found among the DH patients. It is, therefore, possible that a gene dosage effect of DQB1*02 may be present also in DH patients.

DH and CD both are primarily associated with the same DQ ($\alpha1*0501$, $\beta1*02$) heterodimers, and in both diseases most of the few remaining patients not carrying this heterodimer instead carry the DQ ($\alpha1*03$, $\beta1*0302$) heterodimers.

In patients where a jejunal biopsy has been performed have been detected abnormal biopsies both among the DQ ($\alpha1*0501$, $\beta1*02$) positive and negative patients. No significant differences in the frequency of abnormal biopsies were observed between the two groups of patients.

CD and DH have different HLA associations; CD being primarily associated with genes in the DQ/DR region, while DH was more strongly associated with genes in the complement region. Anyway, the very similar associations in CD and DH to the same cis or trans associated DQ2 heterodimer, or the DQ8 heterodimer, can be taken as an argument against differences in primary HLA associations in these two diseases [41].

12. HLA DQ2 in recurrent pregnancy loss women

Recurrent pregnancy loss (RPL) is diagnosed when three or more consecutive spontaneous abortions occur. RPL occurs in about 2–3% of clinically diagnosed pregnancies of reproductive-aged women.

At present, accepted etiologies for RPL include parental chromosomal abnormalities, untreated hypothyroidism, uncontrolled diabetes mellitus, certain uterine anatomic abnormalities, antiphospholipid antibody syndrome, thrombophilias, infections, and environmental factors [42].

In RPL women, an increased risk of immune abnormalities, such as increased antinuclear antibodies (ANA) and thyroid antibody is been observed [43].

However, in 40% of cases, the cause is unknown.

A significant association between RPL and celiac disease is been demonstrated. Various pathogenic mechanisms underlying the pregnancy failure in CD have been suggested: among them the ability of anti-transglutaminase antibodies to impair the trophoblast invasiveness and endometrial endothelial cells differentiation and disrupt early placentation. A higher proportion of individuals HLA DQ2/DQ8 positive in women with RPL compared to controls is found, (52.6% vs. 23.6%), with 3.6 times higher odds of DQ2/DQ8 positivity.

Whether a similar mechanism to that of CD can be linked to this obstetric complication needs to be investigated. This model might appear a simplification of all the complex mechanisms underlying RPL.

The HLA-DQ2/DQ8 alleles by themselves, outside of CD, are found more frequently in RPL women. A possible pathogenic link of HLA-DQ2/DQ8 positivity, in presence of exogenous still unknown stimuli, may favor an immune condition with detrimental effects during the early stages of pregnancy.

A statistically significant association between HLA-DQ2/DQ8 and ANA positivity in RPL women is demonstrated. There is a significantly higher prevalence of ANA positivity in RPL women compared to control (~ 50% vs. 8.3%–27%).

ANA are a group of autoantibodies found both in the serum of patients with autoimmune and rheumatic diseases and in the general population.

As serological markers, ANA show diagnostic and prognostic significance, while their clinical utility in normal individuals is still unclear. Even if many serologically positive individuals will never develop an autoimmune disease, others may be in a pre-autoimmune state.

Further studies are needed to better understand the possible pathogenic mechanism to this observation; the clinical and therapeutic implications of our observation to provide a new approach to RPL couples [44].

13. HLA-DQ2 and allergy

HLA class-II alleles are associated with some allergies indicating that these alleles might confer susceptibility to the respective allergens. HLA plays a role in antigen/allergen presentation and IgE deregulations.

Few studies have associated HLA DQ2/DQ8 with allergy and other ones have analyzed the association between HLA class II antigens and the specific IgE response to purified allergens. One of these studies found an association between DQ8 and have in specific IgE immune response in individuals with a latex allergy, while others found DQ2 to be associated with olive pollen. However, the association of HLA DQ2/8 with allergy remains unclear.

There is a significant difference between HLA DQ2/8-positive and -negative individuals for dust mite allergy.

A significant association between the IgE antibody response to a highly purified allergen from olive tree pollen and HLA class II antigens DR7 and DQ2 in Spanish patients with seasonal allergic pollenosis is reported. The HLA-DQ2 phenotypic frequency is greater in patients with IgE antibodies olive tree pollen compared with the control group.

The combined involvement of DR and DQ in the allergen response has only been described in the study of reactive T-cell repertoire in a mite sensitized patient. It's identified HLA-DR and DQ restricted T-cell epitopes, one of which can bind to both DR and DQ molecules.

These results empathize the importance of genetic factors in the allergic response. As described in several reports, antigen-specific and non-specific factors are involved in genetic restriction.

Until now none of these factors can be considered as the exclusive determinant of the restriction. It is necessary to perform more studies with T-cell lines and peptides of this protein to determine which is the main region implicated in this response, and clarify this complex response [45].

14. HLA-DQ2 and HIV

Infection with human immunodeficiency virus type 1 (HIV-1) and progression to acquired immune deficiency syndrome (AIDS) are controlled by both host genetic factors and viral factors.

The HLA region controls immune response functions and tissue rejection and influences susceptibility to infectious diseases including HIV. There are HLA class II alleles associated with susceptibility to and protection from HIV-1 infection and that these differences between ethnic groups.

In the HIV+ Caucasian group, a poor prognosis was associated with HLA-DQ2 and a preferable prognosis was associated with HLA-DQ3.

The HLA-DQ3 association appears to be linked with the development of Toxoplasmic Encephalitis (TE) in AIDS. An association of HLA-DQ2 with the occurrence of opportunistic infections in AIDS patients is been confirmed [46]. Of interest was the absence of difference in the frequencies of the HLA-DQ2 antigen between TE patients and controls.

The development of TE in HIV infected patients is regulated by genes in or near the HLA complex and suggests that HLA-DQ typing may help in decisions regarding TE prophylaxis.

An immune response gene in the DQ region may control the progression of HIV infection in adults. The rapidly progressive DQ-associated peptide might block the progression of HIV if given as a novel vaccine [47].

15. HLA-DQ2 and vaccines

Although DQ2 is associated with vigorous antigluten T cell responses, DQ2 also is associated with poor responses to several vaccines and failure to control hepatitis virus C and hepatitis virus B.

Studies analyses the association between HLA class II alleles and haplotypes with antibody response to recombinant HBsAg vaccination in Iranian healthy adult individuals. The results, in parallel with other reports, confirm the association of certain HLA class-II alleles with a lack of antibody response to HBsAg vaccine [48].

Discordant HLA/peptide binding and cytokine production patterns observed in genetically identical monozygotic twins vaccinated with HBsAg suggest the involvement of post genetic and environmental factors influencing the T cell repertoire.

However, APC from non-responders can present HBsAg to HLA class II-matched T-cells of responders. This indicates that defective HBsAg-specific T-cell repertoire rather than APC dysfunction could be involved in vaccination failure [49].

Several studies have established significant associations between DQ2, primary sclerosing cholangitis, and hepatitis C virus recurrence after transplant. A significant relationship between the individual scores of HLA mismatches HLA-DQ2 and the recurrence of HCV was observed.

The large proportion of DQ2/8 positive viral hepatitis patients agrees with the hypothesis that these haplotypes may be involved in certain liver disease pathogenesis. DR3-DQ2 haplotype is the principal risk factor for the disease [50].

Analyses by restriction fragment length polymorphism do not implicate a single susceptibility gene at the DQ locus. The unique factor that allows patients with autoimmune hepatitis to be distinguished from normal subjects or those with viral hepatitis is the DR3-DQ2 haplotype.

The association of DQ2 with suboptimal responses to some viruses raised the possibility that its reduced interaction with DM might also lead to the presentation of moderate-affinity viral peptides, whose unstable binding to DQ2 would reduce the surface of the DQ2/peptide complex and compromise CD4+ T cell responses [51].

16. HLA-DQ2 and autism

HLA genes also play a role in reproduction, pregnancy maintenance, in parental recognition and have been associated with over 100 diseases and disorders including autism.

Autism remained a poorly understood pathology for several decades. It is important to note that the diagnostic criteria have been modified over the years to include a broader category of symptoms, thus increasing the number of children diagnosed with the disorder, now referred to as Autism Spectrum Disorder (ASD) [52].

It has been reported that ASD subjects often have associations with HLA genes or haplotypes, suggesting underlying deregulation of the immune system mediated by HLA genes.

A significant number of autistic children have serum levels of IgA antibodies against the enzyme tissue transglutaminase II (TG2) above normal, and the expression of these antibodies is linked to the HLA-DR3, DQ2, and DR7, DQ2 haplotypes [53].

TG2 is expressed in the brain, where it is important in cell adhesion and synaptic stabilization.

These children constitute a subpopulation of autistic children who fall within the autism disease spectrum, and for whom autoimmunity may represent a significant etiological component of their autism.

17. HLA-DQ2 and multiple sclerosis

Multiple sclerosis is a chronic disease in young adults. It is caused by the demyelination of the central nervous system cells. It is considered a T-cell-mediated autoimmune disease that is likely caused by exogenous events, such as infectious agents, in susceptible individuals [54].

Population, family, and twin studies indicate that genetic factors and most likely several genes are associated with the disease, but genetic backgrounds as well as exogenous or somatic events are required to develop the disease. The strongest genetic association with disease among the many candidate genes that were analyzed was demonstrated for HLA-DR15, HLA-DQ2, and HLA-DQ6 [55]. HLA-class II haplotypes such as DR2/DQ6, DR3/DQ2, and DR4/DQ8 show the strongest linkage with the disease.

A positive connection of primary progressive MS with DR4-DQ8 and DR1-DQ5 and an association of "bout onset" MS with DR17-DQ2 is be found, while an HLA association with disease severity was not found [56].

It is currently unclear how the expression of a particular HLA class II gene would result in susceptibility to develop an organ-specific autoimmune disease.

18. HLA-DQ2 and world frequencies

The HLADQ2 associated disease risk is known to be modified across individuals or populations varying in ethnic background, geography, or gender.

The presence of genes coding for DQ2 and DQ8 molecules explains up to 40% of the occurrence of celiac disease in European populations. DQ2 is most common in Western Europe; higher frequencies are observed in parts of Spain and Ireland. In European celiac patients, the frequency of the HLA DQ2 is up by 90% e the HLA DQ8 is between five and 10% like was described in Dutch, UK, and Irish cases.

Differences in the frequencies of the HLA genotypes DQ2 and DQ8 in non-European populations have already been described. Patients of Indian origin had a lower frequency of HLA DQ2 than those of British origin. Lower frequencies of HLA DQ2 and higher frequency of HLA DQ8 than Europe have also been described among CD patients in the United States (82% DQ2 and 16% DQ8 only) and in Cuba (86% DQ2) In Chilean celiac patients the genotype DQ8 predominates. The genotypes

DQ2 and DQ8 were present in 93.2% of patients with CD in the Northeast of Brazil. The HLA DQ2 was present in 75.6% and DQ8 in 17.8% of these patients.

Another finding from this group is that 79% of the unaffected control families carried genotype DQ2 and/or DQ8, which is one of the highest frequencies so far described among first-degree relatives. Most studies on HLA among first-degree relatives found that no more than 59.5% of first-degree relatives in Europe presented HLA DQ2 and DQ8. Since the frequencies of genetic markers among populations of first-degree relatives reflect and amplify those among the general population of which they form part, in this region, a large proportion of the general population may carry these markers.

The frequencies of the different isoforms of DQ2 were also analyzed. The Eurasian geographic distribution of DQ2.2 is slightly greater than DQ2.5. Compared to DQ2.5, the frequency in Sardinia is low, but in Iberia, it is high reaching a maximum frequency of ~30% in Northern Iberia, and half that in the British.

Cases of DQ2.2 patients with CD without DQ2.5 are in some populations, particularly in the south of Europe. It extends along the Mediterranean and Africa at relatively high frequency and is found in high frequencies in some Central Asian, Mongolians, and Han Chinese. It does not appear to have an indigenous presence in the West Pacific Rim and DQ2.2 presence in South-east Asia and Indonesia is likely the result of gene flow from India and China in the past. The haplotype shows considerable diversity in Africa. The expansion of DQ2.2 into Europe appears to have been slightly later. DQ2.5 is generally highest in northern, Icelandic Europe, and Basque in northern Spain. Phenotype frequency exceeds 50% in parts of Ireland, which overlaps one of three global nodes of the DQ2.5 haplotype in Western Europe [57].

19. Conclusion

This work is designed to provide a quick overview of the HLA-DQ2 molecule, analyzing the main points such as molecular structure, gene variants, and the role played by the molecule in the clinical context; dealing not only with the most known autoimmune diseases to which it is linked but also with less known areas of development.

This work aimed to offer a new point of view on the subject, although aware of having only skimmed the topic, we hope to have offered a starting point for any new analysis of the molecule.

This chapter allowed us to analyze HLA in a different context from the most known of compatibility in hematopoietic stem cell transplantation, confirming once again the enormous complexity of the HLA system and its many facets and applications.

Author details

Federica Gualandris[1]*, Laura Castellani[2] and Anna Falanga[3]

1 ASST Papa Giovanni XXIII UOC Immunoematologia e Medicina Trasfusionale (SIMT), Laboratorio di Immunogenetica, Bergamo, Italy

2 ASST Papa Giovanni XXIII UOC Immunoematologia e Medicina Trasfusionale (SIMT), Laboratorio di Immunogenetica Director, Bergamo, Italy

3 Università Milano Bicocca, Dipartimento di Medicina e Chirurgia; ASST Papa Giovanni XXIII UOC Immunoematologia e Medicina Trasfusionale (SIMT) Director, Bergamo, Italy

*Address all correspondence to: federicagualandris.fg@gmail.com

IntechOpen

References

[1] https://www.immunopaedia. org.za/immunology/ basics/4-mhc-antigen-presentation/

[2] Bellanti, JA (Ed). Immunology IV: Clinical Applications in Health and Disease. I Care Press, Bethesda, MD, 2012

[3] Bellanti, JA (Ed). Immunology IV: Clinical Applications in Health and Disease. I Care Press, Bethesda, MD, 2012

[4] Structural and functional studies of trans encoded HLA-DQ2.3. Stig Tollefsen, Kinya Hotta, Xi Chen, Bjørg Simonsen, Kunchithapadam Swaminathan, Irimpan I. Mathews, Ludvig M. Sollid, and Chu-Young Kim, J Biol Chem. 2012 Apr 20; 287(17): 13611-13619. Published online 2012 Feb 23. doi: 10.1074/jbc.M111.320374

[5] Wikipedia: HLA-DQ2

[6] HLA types in celiac disease patients not carrying the DQA1*05-DQB1*02 (DQ2) heterodimer: results from the European Genetics Cluster on Celiac Disease; Kati Karell 1, Andrew S Louka, Simon J Moodie, Henry Ascher, Fabienne Clot, Luigi Greco, Paul J Ciclitira, Ludvig M Sollid, Jukka Partanen, European Genetics Cluster on Celiac Disease; May 2003 Human Immunology 64(4):469-77 DOI: 10.1016/S0198-8859(03)00027-2

[7] What-when-how In Depth Tutorials and Information The Major Histocompatibility Complex (The Immune System in Health and Disease) (Rheumatology) Part 2

[8] The peptide-binding motif of the disease-associated HLA-DQ (alpha 1* 0501, beta 1* 0201) molecule F Vartdal 1, B H Johansen, T Friede, C J Thorpe, S Stevanović, J E Eriksen, K Sletten, E Thorsby, HG Rammensee, L M Solid; Eur J Immunol 1996 Nov;26(11):276472. doi:10.1002/eji.1830261132.

[9] Crystal structure of HLA-DQ2.5-CLIP1 at 2.73 resolutions DOI: 10.2210/ pdb5KSU/PDB

[10] Peptide binding characteristics of the coeliac disease-associated DQ (alpha1*0501, beta1*0201) molecule. van de Wal Y, Kooy YM, Drijfhout JW, Amons R, Koning F Immunogenetics. 1996; 44(4):246-53.

[11] The peptide-binding motif of the disease-associated HLA-DQ (alpha 1* 0501, beta 1* 0201) molecule. Vartdal F, Johansen BH, Friede T, Thorpe CJ, Stevanović S, Eriksen JE, Sletten K, Thorsby E, Rammensee HG, Solid LM Eur J Immunol. 1996 Nov; 26(11):2764-72.

[12] Tissue transglutaminase selectively modifies gliadin peptides that are recognized by gut-derived T cells in celiac disease. Molberg O, Mcadam SN, Körner R, Quarsten H, Kristiansen C, Madsen L, Fugger L, Scott H, Norén O, Roepstorff P, Lundin KE, Sjöström H, Solid LM Nat Med. 1998 Jun; 4(6):713-7.

[13] Different binding motifs of the celiac disease-associated HLA molecules DQ2.5, DQ2.2, and DQ7.5 revealed by relative quantitative proteomics of endogenous peptide repertoires Elin Bergseng 1, Siri Dørum, Magnus Ø Arntzen, Morten Nielsen, Ståle Nygård, Søren Buus, Gustavo A de Souza, Ludvig M Solid Immunogenetics 2015 Feb;67(2):73-84. doi: 10.1007/s00251-014-0819-9. Epub 2014 Dec 12.

[14] Specificity of tissue transglutaminase explains cereal toxicity in celiac disease. Vader LW, de Ru A, van der Wal Y, Kooy YM, Benckhuijsen W, Mearin ML, Drijfhout JW, van Veelen P, Koning F J Exp Med. 2002 Mar 4; 195(5):643-9.

[15] Crystal structure of HLA-DQ2.2-glut-L1 (protein) resolutions DOI: 10.2210/pdb5KSU/PDB

[16] A molecular basis for the T cell response in HLA-DQ2.2 mediated celiac disease Yi Tian Ting, View ORCID ProfileShiva Dahal-Koirala, Hui Shi Keshia Kim, Shuo-Wang Qiao, Ralf S. Neumann, Knut E. A. Lundin, Jan Petersen, Hugh H. Reid, Ve Ludvig M. Sollid, and Jamie Rossjohn PNAS February 11, 2020, 117 (6) 3063-3073; first published January 23, 2020; https://doi.org/10.1073/pnas.191430811

[17] T-Cell Response to Gluten in Patients With HLA-DQ2.2 Reveals Requirement of Peptide-MHC Stability in Celiac DiseaseMichael BoddChu–Young KimKnut E.A. LundinLudvig M. Sollid Gastroenterology 2012 Mar;142(3):552-61.doi: 10.1053/j.gastro.2011.11.021. Epub 2011 Nov 19

[18] Structural and functional studies of the trans-encoded HLA-DQ2.3 (DQA1*03:01/DQB1*02:01) molecule DOI: 10.2210/pdb4D8P/pdb

[19] https://www.euroimmun.it/prodotti/biologia-molecolare/hla-dq2-dq8/

[20] Celiac Disease Ludvig M. Sollid, Knut E.A. Lundin, in The Autoimmune Diseases (Fifth Edition), 2014

[21] Genotype DQ2.5/DQ2.2 (ββ2/ββ2) and High Celiac Disease Risk Development; Yanna Karla de Medeiros Nóbrega; November 30th 2018; DOI: 10.5772/intechopen.80578

[22] T cell sensing of antigen dose governs interactive behavior with dendritic cells and sets a threshold for T cell activation. Henrickson S.E.Mempel T.R. Mazo I.B. et al. 9 Fallang L.E. Bergseng E. Hotta K. et al. Nat Immunol. 2008; 9: 282-291

[23] A molecular basis for the T cell response in HLA-DQ2.2 mediated celiac disease Yi Tian Ting, Shiva Dahal-Koirala, Hui Shi Keshia Kim, Shuo-Wang Qiao, Ralf S. Neumann, Knut E. A. Lundin, Jan Petersen, Hugh H. Reid, Ludvig M. Sollid, and Jamie Rossjohn PNAS February 11, 2020, 117 (6) 3063-3073; first published January 23, 2020; https://doi.org/10.1073/pnas.191430811

[24] Cellular and Molecular Immunology; Abbas & Lichman; Elsevier 2005. 5e www.studentconsult.com

[25] Epitope Selection for HLA-DQ2 Presentation: Implications for Celiac Disease and Viral Defense; Shu-Chen Hung, Tieying Hou, Wei Jiang, Nan Wang, Shuo-Wang Qiao, I-Ting Chow, Xiaodan Liu, Sjoerd H. van der Burg, David M. Koelle, William W. Kwok, Ludvig M. Sollidand Elizabeth D. Mellins, J Immunol May 1, 2019, 202 (9) 2558-2569; DOI: https://doi.org/10.4049/jimmunol.1801454

[26] Classification and Management of Refractory Celiac Disease Alberto Rubio-Tapia, MD and Joseph A Murray, MD PMC 2011 Apr 1. Gut. 2010 Apr; 59(4): 547-557. doi: 10.1136/gut.2009.195131

[27] HLA genotyping in pediatric celiac disease patients Biljana Stanković, Nedeljko Radlović, Zoran Leković, Dragana Ristić, Vladimir Radlović, Gordana Nikčević, Nikola Kotur, Ksenija Vučićević, Tatjana Kostić, Sonja Pavlović, and Branka Zukić, Bosn J Basic Med Sci. 2014 Aug; 14(3): 171-176. doi: 10.17305/bjbms.2014.3.28

[28] Whole-Genome Analysis and HLA Genotyping of Enteropathy-Type T-Cell Lymphoma Reveals 2 Distinct Lymphoma Subtypes; Ronald J Deleeuw , Andreas Zettl, Erdwine Klinker, Eugenia Haralambieva, Magan Trottier, Raj Chari, Yong Ge, Randy D Gascoyne, Andreas Chott, Hans-Konrad Müller-Hermelink, Wan L Lam Gastroenterology 2007

May;132(5):1902-11. doi: 10.1053/j. gastro.2007.03.036. Epub 2007 Mar 24.

[29] Human Leukocyte Antigen-DQ2 Homozygosity and the Development of Refractory Celiac Disease and Enteropathy-Associated T-Cell Lymphoma Abdulbaqi Al Toma, Marije S. Goerres, Jos W. R. Meijer, A. Salvador Peña , J. Bart, A. Crusius, and Chris J. J. Mulder; Clin Gastroenterol Hepatol 2006 Mar;4(3):315-9. doi: 10.1016/j.cgh.2005.12.011.

[30] The HLA-DQ2 gene dose effect in celiac disease is directly related to the magnitude and breadth of gluten-specific T cell responses Willemijn Vader , Dariusz Stepniak, Yvonne Kooy, Luisa Mearin, Allan Thompson, Jon J van Rood, Liesbeth Spaenij, Frits Koning Proc Natl Acad Sci U S A2003 Oct 14;100(21):12390-5. doi: 10.1073/pnas.2135229100.Epub 2003 Oct 6.

[31] Human leukocyte antigen DQ2/8 prevalence in non-celiac patients with gastrointestinal diseases Daniel DiGiacomo, Antonella Santonicola, Fabiana Zingone, Edoardo Troncone, Maria Cristina Caria, Patrizia Borgheresi, Gianpaolo Parrilli, and Carolina Ciacci; World J Gastroenterol 2013 Apr 28;19(16):2507-13. doi: 10.3748/wjg.v19.i16.2507.

[32] HLA-DQ Genotype Is Associated with Accelerated Small Bowel Transit in Patients with Diarrhea-Predominant Irritable Bowel Syndrome; Maria I Vazquez-Roque 1, Michael Camilleri, Paula Carlson, Sanna McKinzie, Joseph A Murray, Tricia L Brantner, Duane D Burton, Alan R Zinsmeister Eur J Gastroenterol Hepatol 2011 Jun;23(6):481-7. doi: 10.1097/MEG.0b013e328346a56e.

[33] The HLA-DR3, DQ2 heterozygous genotype is associated with an accelerated progression of primary sclerosing cholangitis; K M Boberg, A Spurkland, G Rocca, T Egeland, S

Saarinen, S Mitchell, U Broomé, R Chapman, O Olerup, A Pares, F Rosina, E Schrumpf; Scand J Gastroenterol 2001 Aug;36(8):886-90. doi: 10.1080/003655201750313441.

[34] Thyroid Autoimmunity: Role of Anti-thyroid Antibodies in Thyroid and Extra-Thyroidal Diseases Eleonore Fröhlich1,2 and Richard Wahl; Front Immunol 2017 May 9;8:521. doi: 10.3389/fimmu.2017.00521. e Collection 2017.

[35] Differences in the risk of celiac disease associated with HLA-DQ2.5 or HLA-DQ2.2 are related to sustained gluten antigen presentation. Nat Immunol. 2009; 10: 1096-1101

[36] Etiology of Type 1 Diabetes; John A Todd; April 2010, Immunity 32(4):457-67. DOI: 10.1016/j. immuni.2010.04.001

[37] Genetics of thyroid function and disease Vijay Panicker 1; Clin Biochem Rev 2011 Nov;32(4):165-75.

[38] HLA antigens in Asian Indian patients with Graves' disease; N Tandon 1, N K Mehra, V Taneja, M C Vaidya, N Kochupillai; Clin Endocrinol (Oxf) 1990 Jul;33(1):21-6. doi: 10.1111/j.1365-2265.1990.tb00461.x.

[39] Association of the large multifunctional proteosome (LMP2) gene with Graves' disease is a result of linkage disequilibrium with the HLA haplotype DRB1*0304-DQB1*02-DQA1*0501; J M Heward 1, A Allahabadia, M C Sheppard, A H Barnett, J A Franklyn, S C Goug; Clin Endocrinol (Oxf)1999 Jul;51(1):115-8. doi: 10.1046/j.1365-2265.1999.00755.x.

[40] Dermatitis herpetiformis and celiac disease are both primarily associated with the HLA-DQ (alpha 1*0501, beta 1*02) or the HLA-DQ (alpha 1*03, beta 1*0302) heterodimers; A. Spurdland, G. Ingvarsson, E. S. Falk, 1. Knutsen, L. M.

Sollid, E. Thorsby. Tissue Antigens 1997: 49: 29-34. 0 Munksgaard, 1997

[41] Alterations in HLA-DP and HLA-DQ Antigen Frequency in Patients with Dermatitis Herpetiformis; Russell MartinRene J. Duquesnoy M.D. Stephen I. Katz M.D., Ph.D. J Invest Dermatol1989 Oct;93(4):501-5. doi: 10.1111/1523-1747.ep12284056.

[42] Recurrent Pregnancy Loss: Etiology, Diagnosis, and Therapy; Holly B Ford, MD* and Danny J Schust, MD; Rev Obstet Gynecol Spring 2009;2(2):76-83.

[43] Antiphospholipid Syndrome during pregnancy: the state of the art; Fosca A. F. Di Prima, Oriana Valenti, Entela Hyseni, Elsa Giorgio, Marianna Faraci, Eliana Renda, Roberta De Domenico, and Santo Monte; Journal of Prenatal Medicine; 2011 Apr-Jun; 5(2): 41-53.

[44] Human leukocyte antigen (HLA) DQ2/DQ8 prevalence in recurrent pregnancy loss women; Silvia D'Ippolito, Antonio Gasbarrini, Roberta Castellani , Sandro Rocchetti , Leuconoe Grazia Sisti , Giovanni Scambia, Nicoletta Di Simone; Autoimmun Rev 2016 Jul;15(7):638-43. doi:10.1016/j.autrev.2016.02.009. Epub 2016 Feb 13.

[45] Identification of HLA-DR and -DQ alleles conferring susceptibility to pollen allergy and pollen associated food allergy; Boehncke WH1, Loeliger C, Kuehnl P, Kalbacher H, Böhm BO, Gall H; Clinical and Experimental Allergy : Journal of the British Society for Allergy and Clinical Immunology, 01 Apr 1998, 28(4):434-441; DOI: 10.1046/j.1365-2222.1998.00246.x

[46] Prevalence of toxoplasma encephalitis in AIDS patients treated with Didanosine hospitalised in a French infectious service; Marie-Elisabeth Sarciron , Arnaud Ghérardi, Chantal Delorme, Dominique

Peyramond, Anne-Françoise Pétavy; Curr HIV Res 2004 Oct;2(4):301-7. doi: 10.2174/1570162043351101.

[47] Evidence for Genetic Regulation of Susceptibility to Toxoplasmic Encephalitis in AIDS Patients Yasuhiro Suzuki, Sin-Yew Wong, F. Carl Grumet, Jeffrey Fessel, Jose G. Montoya, Andrew R. Zolopa, Amy Portmore, Francolse Schumacher-Perdreau, Matthias Schrappe, Stefan Koppen,* Bernhard Ruf, Byron William Brown, and Jack S. Remington; J Infect Dis1996 Jan;173(1):265-8. doi: 10.1093/infdis/173.1.265.

[48] HLA-DRB1, DQA1, and DQB1 alleles and haplotypes frequencies in Iranian healthy adult responders and non-responders to recombinant hepatitis B vaccine; Ali Akbar Amirzargar 1, Nilufar Mohseni, Mohammad Ali Shokrgozar, Zohreh Arjang, Nahid Ahmadi, Manijeh Yousefi Behzadi, Amir Amanzadeh, Fazel Shokri; Iran J Immunol 2008 Jun;5(2):92-9.

[49] Humoral response to recombinant hepatitis B virus vaccine at birth: role of HLA and beyond Martinetti, M., A. De Silvestri, C. Belloni, A. Pasi, C. Tinelli, A. Pistorio, L. Salvaneschi, G. Rondini, and M. A. Avanzini. 2000. Clin. Immunol. 97: 234-240.

[50] HLA-DRB1, DQA1, and DQB1 alleles and haplotypes frequencies in Iranian healthy adult responders and non-responders to recombinant hepatitis B vaccine; Amirzargar, A. A., N. Mohseni, M. A. Shokrgozar, Z. Arjang, N. Ahmadi, M. Yousefi Behzadi, A. Amanzadeh, and F. Shokri. 2008. Iran. J. Immunol. 5: 92

[51] Role of HLA allele polymorphism in chronic hepatitis B virus infection and HBV vaccine sensitivity in patients from eastern Turkey; Albayrak, A., M. Ertek, M. A. Tasyaran, and I. Pirim. 2011. Biochem. Genet. 49: 258-269

[52] Advances in Autism;
Daniel H. Geschwind; Annu Rev Med
2009;60:367-80. doi: 10.1146/annurev.
med.60.053107.121225.

[53] Autism spectrum disorders
are associated with an elevated
autoantibody response to tissue
transglutaminase-2; Allen Rosenspire,
Wonsuk Yoo, Sherri Menard,
Anthony R Torres; Autism Res 2011
Aug;4(4):242-9. doi: 10.1002/aur.194.
Epub 2011 Apr 19.

[54] The immunopathogenesis of
multiple sclerosis; Elisabetta Prat,
Roland Martin; J Rehabil Res Dev Mar-
Apr 2002;39(2):187-99.

[55] Genetics of multiple sclerosis-how
could disease-associated HLA-types
contribute to pathogenesis?; Martin R;
J Neural Transm Suppl 1997;49:177-94.
doi: 10.1007/978-3-7091-6844-8_19.

[56] HLA-DRB1*1501, -DQB1*0301,
-DQB1*0302, -DQB1*0602, and
-DQB1*0603 alleles are associated with
more severe disease outcome on Mri
in patients with multiple sclerosis;
Robert Zivadinov 1, Laura Uxa, Alessio
Bratina, Antonio Bosco, Bhooma
Srinivasaraghavan, Alireza Minagar,
Maja Ukmar, Su yen Benedetto, Marino
Zorzon; February 2007 International
Review of Neurobiology 79:521-35 DOI:
10.1016/S0074-7742(07)79023-2

[57] Fequency distribution of HLA DQ2
and DQ8 in celiac patients and first-
degree relatives in Recife, northeastern
Brazil Margarida Maria Castro-Antunes,
Sergio Crovella, Lucas André Cavalcanti
Brandão, Rafael Lima Guimarães, Maria
Eugênia Farias Almeida Motta, and
Giselia Alves Pontes da Silva; Clinics
(Sao Paulo) 2011;66(2):227-31.doi:
10.1590/s1807-59322011000200008.

Chapter 3

Immune Checkpoints as a Novel Source for Diagnostic and Therapeutic Target in Celiac Disease

Isabel Torres, Miguel Ángel López Casado,
Teresa Palomeque and Pedro Lorite

Abstract

Celiac disease, as an autoimmune disorder, is a disease which appears in sensing and immune reaction responses to gluten. It has been confirmed that both genetic and environmental factors are involved. CD is strongly associated with the HLA alleles DQB1*02 (serological DQ2) or DQB1*0302 (serological DQ8). These HLA alleles are necessary but not sufficient for the development of CD and non-HLA risk genes also contribute to disease susceptibility. Several studies have identified linkage or association of CD with the 2q33 locus, a region harboring the candidate genes CD28, CTLA4 and ICOS, important immune checkpoints regulators of T-cell activity. Immune checkpoints are crucial to maintain self-tolerance and protect self-tissue from damage during an ongoing immune response.

Keywords: immune checkpoints, celiac disease, PD1, PDL, HLA-G, CTLA4, IDO, tryptophan

1. Introduction

Celiac disease is a unique autoimmune disorder in that the key genetic components (HLA class II genes DQ2 and/or DQ8) are present in almost all patients, the autoantigen is known (tTG), and, most importantly, the environmental trigger is known (gluten) [1–5]. The HLA-DQ molecules predispose to disease by preferential presentation of gluten antigens to CD4+ T cells [6–8]. These genotypes are necessary for the development of the disease, but they are not the only ones responsible, since these genes are present in the population, and only 1% develop CD [9]. Furthermore, in recent years, other areas of the genome outside the HLA region have also been identified that could influence susceptibility to CD, many are related to immunity, especially with T-cell and B-cell function [10, 11].

Gluten ingestion by patients with CD leads to a cascade of inflammatory reactions and eventually to the hallmark small-intestinal lesion. The most important consequence is reduced nutrient uptake characterized by CD4$^+$ T-cell activation, increasing numbers of intraepithelial lymphocytes with partial to total intestinal villus atrophy [12–15]. A common feature of gluten-derived epitopes is the presence of multiple proline and glutamine residues that are selectively deamidated by tTG.

The passage of immunogenic peptides to the lamina propria stimulates specific CD4 + T lymphocytes when they occur together with HLA-DQ2/DQ8 molecules, after having a modification by tissue transglutaminase (TGt). Proinflammatory cytokine responses are activated and mechanisms causing mucosal alteration. Activation of these gluten-reactive CD4 + T cells lead to a pro-inflammatory response dominated by IFN-γ production [16–18].

The response of CD4 + T cells to post-translationally modified gluten and highly disease specific B cells to deamidated gluten and transglutaminase 2 (TG2) autoprotein are present in the pathogenesis in CD [12]. When immunogenic gluten peptides cross the intestinal lumen, they can trigger an innate and adaptive immune response, leading to the development of clinical and histological manifestations of CD [19].

The immune homeostasis has to be precisely maintained in a physiological state, through a balance of costimulatory (*e.g.* CD28) and coinhibitory (*e.g.* CTLA-4 or PD-1) immune signals known as "immune checkpoints". Immune checkpoints are essential for maintaining self-tolerance, protecting tissues from damage caused by the immune system, and providing protective immunity [20]. An imbalance in immune homeostasis can lead to costimulation and the upregulation of T-cell activation in autoimmune diseases [21].

During the normal activation state, CD4$^+$ and CD8$^+$ T cells express multiple immune checkpoint molecules, and some of them also serve a costimulatory function of T cells activation. T cells obtained from individuals with autoimmune conditions have enhanced expression of these molecules that represent an activated T cell state. T lymphocytes play a central role in the induction of an effective adaptive immune response and responsible for maintaining immune homeostasis. Signaling through two well-known negative regulators or checkpoints of T cells, CTLA4 and PD1 leads to direct inhibition of T cell responses [20].

The present chapter discuss the role of the immune checkpoints in intestinal tissue homeostasis and tolerance, and speculate how genetic and environmental factors can regulate them in celiac disease.

2. Immune checkpoints

Immune checkpoints play an essential role in the function and regulation of effector T cells (Teff) and regulator T cells (Treg). Immune checkpoint molecules limits excessive T cell-mediated inflammatory responses and in their signaling processes include a series of ligands that are expressed on the membrane of antigen-presenting cells (APCs) transmitting inhibitory signals (**Figure 1**). These molecules employ specific receptor partners expressed by T lymphocytes and drive their activation and differentiation or promote immunoregulatory effects. Dysregulation of these signaling processes has been associated with autoimmunity and chronic inflammation.

Autoimmune diseases are heterogeneous conditions involving breakdown of tolerance and consequent activation of autoreactive immune cells [22]. The failure of immune checkpoints has been described in inflammatory myopathies with the involvement of autoimmune features [23], as well as in diabetes, multiple sclerosis, systemic lupus erythematosus and celiac disease [24]. Inhibitory checkpoint molecules have been considered as new targets in personalized cancer immunotherapy for their potential in multiple cancer types [21, 25]. An active area of research is the analysis of the functions of these checkpoint molecules and its ligands in tolerance and autoimmunity.

The immune system has the difficult dual function of discerning and defending against a variety of pathogens and avoiding self-reactivity. To further control the

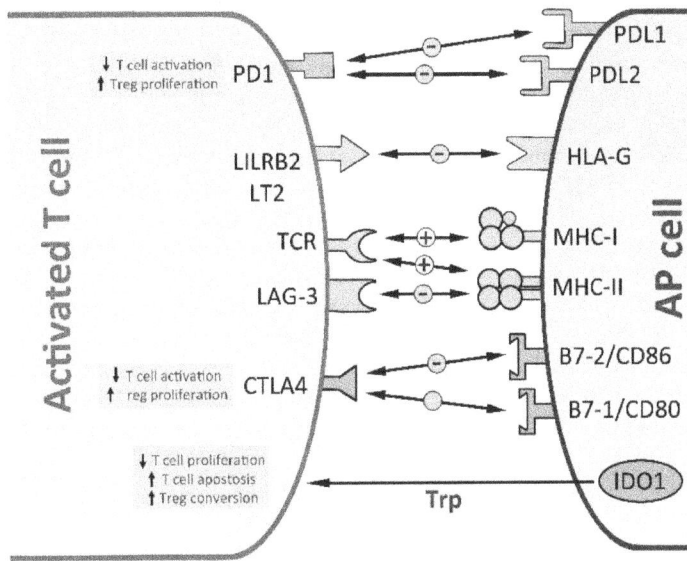

Figure 1.
Schematic representation of immune checkpoint molecules including a series of ligands expressed on the membrane of antigen-presenting cells (APCs), that engage specific receptor partners expressed by T lymphocytes and either drive their activation and differentiation (positive immune checkpoint molecules) or promote immunoregulatory effects (negative immune checkpoint molecules).

development of autoimmunity, multiple mechanisms of peripheral tolerance have evolved, including T-cell anergy, deletion and suppression by Tregs cells. Treg and Teff cells help maintain immune homeostasis through mutual regulation. Loss of homeostatic balance between Teff/Treg cells is often associated with autoimmunity [24, 26].

In this chapter, we will discuss the biology of immune checkpoints, highlight research strategies that may help reduce the incidence of immune related adverse events associated with celiac disease, and also suggest investigational approaches to manipulate immune checkpoints to treat its autoimmune disorder.

2.1 IDO/kynurenine pathway

An important inhibitory checkpoint is now considered to be the tolerogenic mechanism of the enzyme indoleamine-2, 3-dioxygenase (IDO), an intracellular protein involved in the oxidative catabolism of tryptophan (Trp). It catalyzes the conversion of Trp to N-formyl kynurenine via the kynurenine pathway. Depletion of Trp reduces T cell proliferation, whereas the production of kynurenine induces apoptosis of type 1 T helper (Th1) cells and naïve T cell differentiation into Tregs cells [27, 28].

IDO is expressed intracellularly in a constitutive manner in the placenta, epididymis, prostate, esophagus, intestine, colon, cecum, spleen, thymus, lung, brain, and skin [29, 30]. Notably, the morphological features of many IDO-expressing cells closely resemble those of antigen-presenting cells and epithelial cells [29].

IDO expression is inducible by inflammatory stimuli including cytokines and toll like receptor agonists. IDO is expressed in antigen presenting cells, macrophages and dendritic cells, and activation of IDO during the inflammatory response leads to a decrease in local trp levels [27]. These decreased levels have an inhibitory effect on the proliferation of T lymphocytes, directly or indirectly via activation of regulatory T cells [27, 31].

In most cell types, IDO is induced at the transcriptional level in response to specific inflammatory stimuli. IFN-γ is the principal IDO inducer *in vitro* and *in vivo*. Exposure to IFN-γ increases IDO transcription in monocyte/macrophages [32] and dendritic cells [33], fibroblasts [34], epithelial cells [35], smooth muscle cells [36]. Other inflammatory stimuli, such as IFN-α, IFN-β, LPS and cytotoxic T lymphocyte-associated antigen (CTLA)-4, also induce IDO to a lesser degree than that of IFN-γ [37, 38].

A dysfunctional IDO has recently been associated with a specific single nucleotide polymorphism (SNP) and with the occurrence of autoimmune diabetes and multiple sclerosis. The elevated levels of kynurenines that are present contain the proliferation of Teff cells and favor the differentiation of Treg cells [39]. Several genetic variations of the *IDO* gene have been associated with the occurrence and severity of autoimmune/chronic inflammatory diseases; however, the functional relevance of these variations, which mainly affect the intron regions and the promoter portion of IDO, has not been well characterized yet [40, 41].

In celiac disease, mechanisms dependent on tryptophan catabolism may be involved in the regulation of the immune response. Thus, in intestinal biopsies from celiac patients, a high expression of the anti-inflammatory enzyme IDO appears [42]. This increase in IDO levels results in an increase in serum levels of kynurenine in patients with celiac disease, which potentially contributes to intensify inflammation. Likewise, higher levels of kynurenine were found in celiac patients with other associated diseases, such as Down syndrome or autoimmune thyroiditis, contributing to the pathology [43].

Once an autoimmune disorder is established, the presence of chronic inflammation might provoke sustained IDO production and IDO fails to limit immune deregulation under these pathological conditions. Several inflammatory mediators including the most potent, IFN-γ, induce IDO production. Wolf *et al*. [44], have described overexpression of IDO in other Th1-associated chronic inflammatory disease of the gastrointestinal tract, such as Crohn's disease, with increased kynurenine levels and a higher kynurenine/tryptophan ratio. In this pathology has been demonstrated that T helper 1 (Th1)-like cytokines such as IFN-γ and TNF-α are potent inducers of IDO expression.

2.2 HLA-G/ILT interaction is an immune checkpoint

The *HLA-G* gene is a non-classical class I HLA composed of eight exons and seven introns located on chromosome 6 at region 6p21.3, [45]. As a result of alternative RNA splicing, seven isoforms can be formed, comprising four membrane-bound isoforms (HLA-G1, G2, G3, and G4), and three secreted soluble isoforms (HLA-G5, G6, and G7) [46, 47]. Most studies focus on the full-length molecule (HLA-G1) and its soluble isoform (HLA-G5). These isoforms are identical, except HLA-G5 is missing the transmembrane domain.

HLA-G is considered to be an immune checkpoint molecule, a function that is closely linked to the structure and dynamics of the different HLA-G isoforms. The expression of HLA-G can be induced in several conditions, including cancer, transplantation, viral infections, and autoimmune and inflammatory diseases [48–51].

HLA-G mediates its function by binding to receptors on immune cells. The known receptors are leukocyte Ig-like receptor subfamily B member 1 (LILRB1) and member 2 (LILRB2), also known as ILT2 and ILT4, and the killer immunoglobulin-like receptor 2DL4 (KIR2DL4) [52]. ILT2 is expressed by B cells, some subtypes of T cells and NK cells, and all monocytes/dendritic cells. On the other hand, ILT4 is myeloid-specific and only expressed by monocytes/dendritic cells [53].

HLA-G expression and gene polymorphisms have been associated with several disorders [54–56]. HLA-G has an important role in regulating the immune system;

indeed, the molecule is able to inhibit the cytotoxic activity of Natural Killer cells (NK) and T cell-mediated cytolysis (CTL) [57]. HLAG can inhibit the response of alloproliferative CD4+ T cells, proliferation of T and NK cells, and the maturation and function of antigen presenting cells (APC) [58, 59]. In addition, HLA-G has a tolerogenic effect due to its capacity of generating suppressor cells by binding to specific receptors and it can induce apoptosis in endothelial cells [60].

The soluble form of HLA-G is of special interest in celiac disease because its molecule plays an important role in the induction of immune tolerance [61]. In this sense, soluble HLA-G has the function to inhibit the proliferation of activated T cells, and to induce apoptosis of T cells dose dependently, reinforcing the immune inhibitory role of soluble HLA-G capable to be secreted during CD as part of a mechanism to restore the tolerance process towards oral antigens [61, 62]. A potent anti-inflammatory response to gliadin may occur during disease development as a result of the adaptive response in CD. In celiac patients, gluten intake appears to cause an overreaction in intraepithelial T lymphocytes, with uncontrolled production of the HLA-G molecule [61]. This can cause the recruitment of intraepithelial lymphocytes, leading to amplified immune activity and maintenance of intestinal lesions. The increased expression of the soluble form of HLA-G in patients with CD could be part of a mechanism to restore gluten tolerance [61, 62].

Moreover, an association between HLA-G polymorphism and CD has already been described by Fabris et al. [63]. The 14 bp inserted (I) allele and the homozygous I/I genotype were significantly more frequent in CD patients than in healthy controls. The effect of the HLA-G D/I polymorphism is restricted for HLA-DQ2, and not simply due to the presence of linkage disequilibrium with the major known risk factor. In this sense, the risk conferred by HLA-DQ2 alone and that subjects that carry both DQ2 and HLA-G I alleles have an increased risk of CD than subjects that carry DQ2 but not the 14 bp inserted (I) allele [63]. The modulation of the HLA-G transcript stability is especially known for the 14 bp D/I polymorphism, which has been associated with autoimmunity [64–67]. Based on the findings of Torres et al. [61] and considering that the presence of HLA-G SNPs affect the mRNA stability in CD patients, lower basal levels of HLA-G molecule, possibly due to the presence of genetic variations, can increase the risk of celiac disease development. Once that the disease has occurred the organism produces higher levels of soluble HLA-G trying to restore the immune tolerance [61, 62]. Similarly to 5'URR, also 3'UTR presents numerous polymorphic sites that could affect HLA-G transcription and/or translation [68]. By sequencing this region, there are 4 polymorphisms showing some significant associations with CD [64].

In summary, it has been shown that both HLA-G and IDO suppressor molecules are expressed in CD. The expression of these molecules, IDO and HLA-G, would be an essential mechanism to try to restore tolerance towards antigens in the diet [61, 62]. Therefore, the increase in IDO activity reflects an attempt to control chronic antigenic stimulation by downregulating the T cell-mediated autoimmune reaction. IDO and HLA-G could cooperate to suppress the immune response in CD in their active form [61].

López *et al.* [69] showed that suppressive molecules IDO and HLA-G are both expressed in dendritic cells, and these molecules can produce immunosuppression. Besides, IDO was shown to induce HLA-G expression during monocyte differentiation into DCs [69]. IDO and HLA-G share some properties: both have tolerogenic capacity, are highly expressed in human placenta and tumors [70, 71] and their expression can be regulated by the same cytokines (IFN-γ, IL-10) [72, 73]. The effect of IDO on HLA-G cell-surface expression seemed to be dependent on the type of cell studied and is likely to involve posttranslational mechanisms [74]. The inhibition of IDO function with 1-methyl tryptophan in antigen-presenting cells (APCs), which are originally HLA-G cell-surface negatives, increases the levels of

HLA-G1 cell-surface expression, whereas high concentrations of tryptophan caused a loss of HLA-G1 expression in HLA-G1-positive cells [75].

2.3 CD28/CTLA4-B7 pathway

The immune regulatory proteins cytotoxic T lymphocyte antigen (CTLA-4) is important immune regulatory protein collectively referred to as immune check-point receptor. CTLA-4 is known to be crucial for tolerance induction in the early stages of the immune response being an important negative regulator of T-cell activation and proliferation, interacting with B7 molecules on antigen-presenting cells [76, 77]. The *CTLA4* gene encodes a receptor involved in the control of T-cell proliferation and mediates T-cell apoptosis. *CTLA-4* is therefore a plausible candidate for a susceptibility gene in diseases with T-cell mediated pathogenesis [77].

The chromosomal region 2q33 contains immunologically important genes, CD28 and ICOS, that has been associated with autoimmune disease, but the exact causal genetic sequence variation has yet to be established in CD [78]. There is good evidence that the *CTLA-4* region on chromosome 2q33 contains a non-HLA susceptibility locus for celiac disease, although its participation may vary according to the geographic origin of the patients [79]. The association of several SNPs in the CTLA4 gene with CD, among them, the functional SNP, CT60, suggested that the CT60 polymorphism influences alternate RNA splicing of CTLA4, resulting in differing ratios of a full-length form, flCTLA4, and a soluble form, sCTLA4 of the protein [78].

High levels of serum soluble CTLA-4 in active celiac patients were found and are related to gluten intake. A positive correlation exists between autoantibodies to tissue transglutaminase, the grade of gut mucosa damage and soluble CTLA-4 concentration [80]. This correlation between the amount of serum sCTLA-4 and the grade of gut mucosa damage strongly suggests a possible immunomodulatory effect of this soluble molecule on cytotoxic T lymphocyte functions. Thus, soluble CTLA4 appears to be related to autoantibody production per se, independently from dietary gluten [80]. Soluble CTLA-4 could play a critical role in modulating the immune response, especially in the early stage. The immunomodulatory effect of soluble CTLA-4 could be involved in the regulation of B cell activation directly or via T helper function modulation [80].

The detection of the spliced/soluble variant from CD patients suggests that the soluble CTLA-4 does not result from a cleavage of the full-length form [80]. The potential genetic associations of several *CTLA-4* polymorphisms to susceptibility to autoimmune diseases have been described, although the relationship between *CTLA-4* polymorphisms and the ability to produce the soluble form is not fully clarified. CTLA-4 is a strong actor in the adaptive response.

2.4 PD1/PDL pathway

Programmed cell death-1 (PD-1) is a well-established immune checkpoint and co-inhibitory regulator critical to the maintenance of immune tolerance. PD-1 through binding to its PD-L1 and PD-L2 ligands, generate inhibitory signals that regulate the balance between immune system activation, tolerance and immunopathology [81]. The PD1 expression has been noted in activated CD4+/CD8+ T cells, a subset of Tregs, B-cells, myeloid DCs, monocytes, exhausted T cells and basal mesenchymal stem cells [82]. Basal levels of expression of ligand PDL1 was observed in mesenchymal stem cells and vascular endothelium. In addition, activated B-cells, DCs and monocytes also express both PD-L1 and PD-L2 [82]. Lower levels of PDL1 expression was reported in unstimulated CD4+/CD8+ T-cells which was increased upon activation.

Cytokines are potent stimuli for PD-L1 and PD-L2 expression. Type 1 and type 2 interferons and TNF-α induce PD-L1 expression in T cells, B cells, endothelial cells, and epithelial cells [83]. IL-2, IL-7, and IL-15 cytokines increase PD-L1 on human T cells. IL-21 can stimulate PD-L1 expression on B cells and IL-10 induces PD-L1 on monocytes. Expression of PD-L2 is stimulated by interferons, IL-4, and GMCSF on dendritic cells *in vitro*, and the common γ chain cytokines can induce PD-L1 and to a lesser extent PD-L2 on human monocytes/macrophages [83].

PD-1 plays a role in differentiating naive T cells into Treg cells and can inhibit T-cell responses by developing Treg cells [84]. The PD-1 upregulation is a consequence of the activation of T cells, which is essential to the immune responses. PD-1 expression in Tregs is indispensable for their suppressive functions, and loss of PD1 expression accelerates the generation of Tregs which lose Foxp3 expression and produce pro-inflammatory cytokines and thereby flare autoimmunity [84]. Tregs and the PD-1/ PD-L axis are both critical to immune responses, elimination of either can result in the breakdown of tolerance and the development of autoimmunity. The PD-1/PD-L pathway can prevent autoreactive T cells and protect against autoimmunity. Treg cells induced by the PD-1 pathway can also help maintain immune homeostasis, maintaining the activation threshold for T cells to protect against autoimmunity [81, 82].

Although the PD1 pathway has received considerable attention for its roles in T cell exhaustion and tumor immunosuppression, PD1 cannot be considered a specific molecule for cell exhaustion [85]. In fact, T cells express PD1 during activation, thus being a marker for effector T cells. PD1 is expressed by subsets of tolerant T cells, regulatory T cells, follicular helper T cells, follicular regulatory T cells, and memory T cells. In addition, it is expressed on B cells, NK cells, and some myeloid cells. Expression of PD1 can be found in CD8 + T cells of healthy humans, and these cells do not resemble exhausted T cell populations [85, 86].

Polymorphisms have been described in the gene *Pdcd1* that confer susceptibility to development of autoimmune diseases in humans. Many single nucleotide polymorphisms have been reported and approximately most of them are located in the intron regions of the structural gene [87].

Some of the most studied are the PD-1.1 located in the promoter region, PD-1.2 located in intron 2, PD-1.3 and PD-1.4 located at intron 4, PD-1.9 and PD-1.5 in exon 5 and PD-1.6 at position 32 of the untranslated region. Exist different haplotypes of these SNPs in families Caucasian and it is known that PD-1.1, PD-1.2 and PD-1.9 are in linkage imbalance, while the PD-1.4 and PD-1.5 positions they form a different block [88, 89].

PD1 polymorphisms are associated with susceptibility to a variety of autoimmune conditions including systemic lupus erythematosus, rheumatoid arthritis, and progression in multiple sclerosis [89], but it is not yet clear if these SNPs are causative or simply correlative. Furthermore, autoantibodies against PDL1 have been found in patients with rheumatoid arthritis and correlate with disease activity [89].

Ponce de León et al. [90] have focused the alteration of PD-1/PD-L1 pathway in celiac disease. Levels of sPD-1 was considerably higher in the serum of patients with celiac disease compared with health controls. A negative expression of PD1 in intestinal epithelial cells and lamina propria cells of active CD patients. PD-1 protein expression in CD4 + and CD8 + T cells decreases significantly in patients with CD. In this way, PD-1 function would be compromised in CD4 + and CD8 + T cells, indicating an inappropriate activation state [90]. In CD, a deregulation of immune suppression mechanisms appears, which can lead to abnormal and persistent activation of T cells and the production of cytokines. Without PD1, excessive immune-mediated tissue damage can lead to devastating consequences, because PD1 plays crucial roles in central and peripheral T cell tolerance, aiding in the protection of self-tissues from autoimmune responses. The co-delivery of soluble PD-1 could increase the maturation of DCs, which could accompanied by upregulation of DC maturation markers such as major histocompatibility complex II (MHC II) [90]. DC maturation is mediated by activated T lymphocytes, therefore sPD-1-regulated DC maturation may be influenced by increased T cell responses [90].

The soluble isoform is likely to have antagonistic effects on PD-1 by interfering with its signaling pathway, particularly considering that PD-1Δ3 still retains the ability to bind to PD-L1/PD-L2 receptors [90]. In patients with CD, excessive soluble PD-1 could serve as an "antibody" to block the PD-1/PD-Ls pathway and lead to aberrant T-cell proliferation. If, for example, CD8 + T-cell responses are not adequately controlled, severe immunopathology can result from the production of pro-inflammatory cytokines, such as IFN-γ and TNF-α [91].

Soluble PD-1 can promote T-cell responses through blocking the PD-1/PD-Ls pathway. IFN-γ is crucial for this process but also contributes to the upregulation of PD-L1 which indicates that sPD-1 plays a crucial role not only during the phase of T-cell exhaustion but also during primary T-cell activation and that sPD-1 can be used as an adjuvant to increase T-cell immunity [91, 92]. These findings suggest that at the time of clinical diagnosis of CD, T cells can exhibit features of immune exhaustion. It is not yet known what factor(s) contribute to the dysregulated PD-1 expression and may have increased susceptibility to the autoimmune complications of CD. The PD-1 and PD-L1 levels in the serum and intestinal biopsies of CD patients may be relevant to the determination of a possible correlation between markers of the autoimmune response, inflammation, and disease activity.

3. Future directions

The immune cell activation in the setting of immune checkpoint inhibitors results in unmasking of gluten sensitivity in genetically susceptible people, leading to expansion of previously self-reactive CD4+ T cells and subsequent CD8+ T cell-induced tissue destruction. Soluble immune checkpoint molecules constitute the emerging novel mediators in immune regulation. The relationship between celiac disease and the level of soluble immune checkpoints as sCTLA4, sHLA-G, sPD-1, and sPD-L1 has been shown.

3.1 Immune checkpoints cooperation

The immune checkpoint molecules may be implicated in biological mechanisms underlying celiac disease. Some immune checkpoint molecules serve as inhibitory signaling mediators to maintain immune tolerance, especially in the adaptive immune compartment. There are two forms of these molecules: the surface receptor or membrane-bound and cell-free soluble molecules. The membrane-bound CTLA4, HLA-G, PD-1, PD-L1 regulate T cell homeostasis, inhibit autoreactive T cells, and drive peripheral tolerance in cancer, pregnancy, and sepsis. 12,13 They also promote T regulatory cell development and inhibit the effector T cell differentiation and cytokine production leading to immunosuppression [93]. On the other hand, the soluble forms of these immune checkpoint molecules were discovered later, and their biological functions have gradually been elucidated. The immune regulatory effect of soluble PD-L1, sCTLA-4, and sHLA-G can trigger Treg differentiation and T cells apoptosis due to retention of their receptor [94].

Circulating soluble PD-1, CTLA4 and HLA-G could take part in modulating immune tolerance causing disturbances in the molecular mechanisms responsible for maintenance of balance between effector and regulatory components of the immune system in celiac disease. HLA-G and IDO acting independently, both molecules would be complementary in inducing efficient tolerance status. HLA-G1/HLA-G5 and IDO molecules act on alloreactive T-cell proliferation through two distinct inhibitory pathways. However, as IDO expression is tightly regulated and responsive to inflammatory mediators, HLA-G may indirectly modulate IDO by up-regulating the production of such mediators. For instance, by up-regulating the expression of IL-10, HLA-G may boost the IDO pathway.

The HLA-G/ILT2/ILT4 interactions actually target a broader array of immune effectors than the B7/CTLA4 and PD-1/PD-L1 pathways, since CTLA4 and PD-1 are expressed only on T cells, whereas ILT2 and ILT4 are differentially expressed on NK, T, and B cells as well as monocytes, dendritic cells (DCs), and neutrophils and thus may inhibit the early phases of an immune response (PD-1/PD-L1), or the later phases (B7/CTLA4) [93].

3.2 Gene dysregulation in celiac disease

The detection of the spliced/soluble variant of these immune checkpoints from CD patients suggests that the soluble form of HLA-G, CTLA-4 and PD1 molecules does not result from a cleavage of the full-length form. The potential genetic associations of several polymorphisms to susceptibility to autoimmune diseases have been described, Splicing machinery would act as a biosensor to adapt gene expression to pathophysiological conditions.

Gene dysregulation of these genes could lead to an imbalance in the splice variants present in the cells at any given time. The existence of specific factors in the serum of celiac patients, such as peptides derived from gliadin, would be able to modulate the expression of relevant components of the splice and the function of the splicing machinery. Dietary intervention of gluten peptides can clearly alter the expression pattern of the splicing machinery in humans at risk for CD.

The alternative splicing process may represent a physiological mechanism for maintaining cellular homeostasis, as suggested by different studies that demonstrate that the nutrients can modulate gene expression and, in particular, the splicing of pre-mRNAs that encode regulatory proteins. Minimal disturbances in the alternative splicing process can lead to the generation of deficient proteins that contribute to several human diseases. So, the splicing process may represent an adaptive mechanism in response to different nutritional conditions, and that this mechanism could be in place not only in circulating PBMCs but may also operate in cell types from other tissues and organs tightly coupled to nutrient-dependent metabolic homeostasis, e.g., intestine. So, specifically gluten can modulate processes required for cell homeostasis through the alteration of gene expression and, particularly, the splicing of pre-mRNAs encoding key regulatory proteins.

4. Conclusions

Further investigation on the determination of immunological interactions and biological functions by immune checkpoints in celiac disease is needed to deepen our understanding of the underlying disease mechanism in ourquest for diagnostic and therapeutic target in celiac disease.

Acknowledgements

This work was supported by Research group BIO220, Junta de Andalucía.

Author details

Isabel Torres[1*], Miguel Ángel López Casado[2], Teresa Palomeque[1] and Pedro Lorite[1]

1 Department of Experimental Biology, Campus Universitario Las Lagunillas, Jaén, Spain

2 Departamento de Gastroenterología Pediátrica, Hospital Virgen de las Nieves, Granada, Spain

*Address all correspondence to: mitorres@ujaen.es

IntechOpen

References

[1] Lundin KE, Scott H, Hansen T, Paulsen G, Halstensen TS, Fausa O, Thorsby E, Sollid LM. Gliadin-specific, HLADQ (1*0501 1*0201) restricted T cells isolated from thesmall intestinal mucosa of celiac disease patients. J Exp Med 1993; 178:187-196. DOI: 10.1084/jem.178.1.187

[2] Sollid LM, Jabri B. Triggers and drivers of autoimmunity: lessons from coeliac Disease. Nat Rev Immunol 2013; 13(4): 294-302. DOI: 10.1038/nri3407

[3] Viljamaa M, Kaukinen K, Huhtala H Kyrönpalo S, Rasmussen M, Collin P. Coeliac disease, autoimmune diseases and gluten exposure. Scand J Gastroenterol 2005; 40: 437-443. DOI: 10.1080/00365520510012181

[4] López Casado MA, Lorite P, Ponce de León C, Palomeque T, Torres MI. Celiac disease autoimmunity. Arch Immunol Ther Exp. 2018; 66(6): 423-430. DOI: 10.1007/s00005-018-0520-z

[5] Torres MI, Palomeque T, Lorite P. Celiac disease and other autoimmune disorders. In: Chatzidionysiou K (ed) Autoimmunity pathogenesis, clinical aspects and therapy of specific autoinmune diseases. Intech Croatia. 2015; 131-151. DOI: DOI: 10.5772/60695

[6] Bodd M, Kim CY, Lundin KE, Sollid LM. T-cell response to gluten inpatients with HLA-DQ2.2 reveals requirement of peptide-MHC stability in celiac disease. Gastroenterology. 2012; 142:552-561. DOI: 10.1053/j.gastro.2011.11.021

[7] Hunt KA, Zhernakova A, Turner G Heap GAR, Franke L, Bruinenberg M, et al. Newly identified genetic risk variants for celiac disease related to the immune response. Nat Genet 2008; 40:395-402. DOI: 10.1038/ng.102

[8] Trynka G, Hunt KA, Bockett NA, Romanos J, Mistry V, Szperl A et al. Dense genotying identifies and localizes multiple common and rare variant association signals in celiac disease. Nat Genet 2011; 43:1193-1201. DOI: 10.1038/ng.998

[9] Alaedini A, Green PH. Narrative review: celiac disease: understanding a complex autoimmune disorder. Ann Intern Med 2005; 142: 289-298. DOI: 10.7326/0003-4819-142-4-200502150-00011

[10] Fasano A. Clinical presentation of celiac disease in the pediatric population. Gastroenterology 2005; 128: S68–S73. DOI: 10.1053/j. gastro. 2005 .02.015

[11] Kim CY, Quarsten H, Bergseng E, Khosla C, Sollid LM. Structural basis for HLA-DQ2-mediated presentation of gluten epitopes in celiac disease. Proc Natl Acad Sci USA 2004; 101: 4175-4179. DOI: 10.1073/pnas.0306885101

[12] Torres MI, López Casado MA, Ríos A. New aspects in celiac disease. World J Gastroenterol 2007; 13: 1156-1161. DOI: 10.3748/wjg.v13.i8.1156

[13] Di Sabatino A, Vanoli A, Giuffrida P, Luinetti O, Solcia E, Corazza GR. The function of tissue transglutaminase in celiac disease. Autoimmun Rev 11: 746-753. DOI: 10.1016/j.autrev. 2012.01.007

[14] Sollid LM, Markussen G, Ek J, Gjerde H, Vartdal F, Thorsby E. Evidence for a primary association of celiac disease to a particular HLA-DQ alpha/beta heterodimer. J Exp Med 1989; 169: 345-350. DOI: 10.1084/jem.169.1.345

[15] Anderson RP, Degano P, Godkin AJ. *In vivo* antigen challenge in celiac disease identifies a single

transglutaminase-modified peptide as the dominant A-gliadin T-cell epitope. Nat Med 2000; 6: 337-342. DOI: 10.1038/73200

[16] Jabri B, Kasarda DD, Green PHR. Innate and adaptive immunity: the yin and yang of celiac disease. Immunol Rev 2005; 206: 219-231. DOI: 10.1111/j.0105-2896.2005.00294.x

[17] Sollid LM. Coeliac disease: dissecting a complex inflammatory disorder. Nat Rev Immunol. 2002; 2(9), 647-655. DOI: 10.1038/nri885

[18] Alaedini A, Green PHR. Narrative review: celiac disease: understanding a complex autoimmune disorder. Ann Intern Med. 2005; 142(4), 289-298. DOI: 10.7326 /0003-4819-142-4-200502150-00011

[19] Fasano A, Catassi C. Clinical practice. Celiac disease. N Engl J Med 2012; 367: 2419-26. DOI: 10.1056/ NEJMcp1113994

[20] Orabona C, Mondanelli G, Puccetti P, Grohmann G. Immune Checkpoint Molecules, Personalized Immunotherapy, and Autoimmune Diabetes. Trends Mol Med. 2018, 24 (11): 931-41. Doi: 10.1016/j. molmed.2018.08.005

[21] Calabrese L, Velcheti V. Checkpoint immunotherapy: good for cancer therapy, bad for rheumatic diseases. Ann Rheum Dis 2017; 76: 1-3. DOI: 10.1136/ annrheumdis-2016-209782

[22] Abbas AK, Lohr J, Knoechel B, Nagabhushanam V. T cell tolerance and autoimmunity. Autoimmunity Reviews 2004; 3: 471-475. DOI:10.1016/j.autrev. 2004.07.004

[23] Orabona C, Mondanelli G, Puccetti P, Grohmann G. Immune Checkpoint Molecules, Personalized Immunotherapy, and Autoimmune Diabetes. Trends Mol Med. 2018,

24 (11): 931-41. DOi: 10.1016/j. molmed.2018.08.005

[24] Torres MI, Palomeque T, Lorite P. Celiac Disease and Other Autoimmune Disorders. In: Chatzidionysiou K (ed) Autoimmunity-Pathogenesis, clinical aspects and therapy of specific autoimmune diseases. Intech, Croatia. 2015; 131-151. DOI: 10.5772/60695

[25] Pardoll DM. The blockade of immune checkpoints in cancer immunotherapy, Nat Rev Canc. 2012; 12: 252-264. DOI: 10.1038/nrc3239

[26] Kumar P, Saini S, Khan S, Lele SS, Prabhakar BS. Restoring self-tolerance in autoimmune diseases by enhancing regulatory T-cells. Cell Immunol 2019; 339: 41-49. doi: 10.1016/ j.cellimm.2018.09.008.

[27] Grohmann, U. FallarinoF, Puccetti P. Tolerance, DCs and tryptophan: much ado about IDO. Trends Immunol. 2003; 24: 242-248

[28] Puccetti P, Grohmann U. IDO and regulatory T cells: a role for reverse signalling and non-canonical NF-kappaB acti-vation. Nat Rev Immunol. 2007; 7: 817-823. DOI: 10.1038/nri2163

[29] Dai X, Zhu BT. Indoleamine 2, 3-dioxygenase tissue distribution and cellular localization in mice: implications for its biological functions. J Histochem Cytochem. 2010; 58(1): 17-28. doi: 10.1369/jhc.2009.953604.

[30] Sedlmayr P, Blaschitz A, Wintersteiger R, Semlitsch M, Hammer A, MacKenzie et al. Localization of indoleamine 2, 3-dioxygenase in human female reproductive organs and the placenta. Mol Hum Reprod. 2002; 8(4): 385-391. DOI: 10.1093 /molehr/8.4.385

[31] Mellor AL, Munn DH. Tryptophan catabolism and regulation of adaptive

immunity. J Immunol. 2003; 170: 5809-5813.

[32] Mellor AL, Munn DH. Tryptophan catabolism and T-cell tolerance: immunosuppression by starvation? Immunol Today 1999; 10: 469-473. DOI: 10.1016/s0167-5699(99)01520-0

[33] Mellor AL, Munn DH. IDO expression by dendritic cells: tolerance and tryptophan catabolism. Nat Rev Immunol. 2004; 4: 762-774. DOI: 10.1038 /nri1457

[34] Scheler M, Wenzel J, Tüting T, Takikawa O, Bieber T, Von Bubnoff D. Indoleamine 2,3-Dioxygenase (IDO) : The Antagonist of Type I Interferon-Driven Skin Inflammation?. Am J Pathol. 2007; 171(6): 1936-1943. DOI: 10.2353 /ajpath .2007.070281

[35] Mailankot M, Staniszewska MM, Butler H, Caprara MH, Howell S, Wang B, et al. Indoleamine 2, 3-dioxygenase overexpression causes kynurenine-modification of proteins, fiber cell apoptosis and cataract formation in the mouse lens. Lab Invest. 2009; 89(5):498-512. DOI: 10.1038/ labinvest.2009.22.

[36] Mailankot M, Nagaraj RH. Induction of indoleamine 2, 3-dioxygenase by interferon-gamma in human lens epithelial cells: apoptosis through the formation of 3-hydroxykynurenine. Int J Biochem Cell Biol. 2010; 42(9):1446-54. DOI: 10.1016/j.biocel.2010.04.014

[37] Cuffy MC, Silverio AM, Qin L, Wang Y, Eid R, Brandacher G, et al. Induction of indoleamine 2, 3-dioxygenase in vascular smooth muscle cells by interferon-gamma contributes to medial immunoprivilege. J Immunol. 2007; 179(8): 5246-5254. DOI: 10.4049/jimmunol.179.8.5246

[38] Grohmann U, Orabona C, Fallarino F, Vacca C, Calcinaro F, Falorni A, et al. CTLA-4-Ig regulates tryptophan catabolism in vivo. Nat

Immunol. 2002; 3(11): 1097-1101. DOI: 10.1038/ni846.

[39] Jung ID, Lee CM, Jeong YI, Lee JS, Park WS, Han J, Park YM. Differential regulation of indoleamine 2, 3-dioxygenase by lipopolysaccharide and interferon gamma in murine bone marrow derived dendritic cells. FEBS Lett. 2007; 581(7): 1449-1456. DOI: 10.1016/ j.febslet. 2007.02.073.

[40] Puccetti P, Grohmann U. IDO and regulatory T cells: a role for reverse signalling and non-canonical NF-kappaB activation, Nat Rev Immunol 2007; 7: 817-823 DOI: 10.1038/nri2163

[41] Mondanelli G, Iacono A, Carvalho A, Orabona C, Volpi C, Pallotta MT, et al. Amino acid metabolism as drug target in autoimmune diseases, Autoimmun Rev 2019; 18: 334-348, DOI: 10. 1016/j. autrev.2019.02.004.

[42] Boros FA, Bohár Z, Vécsei L. Genetic alterations affecting the genes encoding the enzymes of the kynurenine pathway and their association with human diseases, Mutat Res. 2018; 776: 32-45. DOI: 10.1016/j.mrrev.2018.03.001

[43] Torres MI, López-Casado MA, Lorite P, Ríos A. Tryptophan metabolism and indoleamine 2,3-dioxygenase expression in coeliac disease. Clin Exp Immunol. 2007; 148(3): 419-424. DOI: 10.1111/j.1365-2249.2007.03365.x

[44] Wolf AM, Wolf D, Rumpold H, Moschen AR, Kaser A, Obrist P et al. Overexpression of indoleamine 2,3-dioxygenase in human inflammatory bowel disease. Clin Immunol. 2004; 113: 47-55. DOI: 10.1016/j.clim.2004.05.004

[45] Klein J, Sato A. The HLA system. First of two parts. N Engl J Med 2000; 343:702-9. DOI: 10.1056/ NEJM200009073431006

[46] Lin A, Yan W-H. Heterogeneity of HLA-G Expression in Cancers: Facing the Challenges. Front Immunol. 2018; 9: 2164. DOI: 10.3389/fimmu.2018.02164

[47] Paul P, Cabestre F, Ibrahim E, Lefebvre S, Khalil-Daher I, Vazeux G, et al. Identification of HLA-G7 as a New Splice Variant of the HLA-G mRNA and Expression of Soluble HLA-G5, –G6, and -G7 Transcripts in Human Transfected Cells. Hum Immunol 2000; 61: 1138-1149 (2000). DOI: 10.1016/S0198-8859(00)00197-X

[48] Rouas-Freiss N, Moreau P, Ferrone S, Carosella ED. HLA-G Proteins in Cancer: Do They Provide Tumor Cells with an Escape Mechanism? Cancer Res. 2005; 65(22): 10139-10144. DOI: 10.1158/ 0008-5472.CAN-05-0097

[49] Lila N, Carpentier A, Amrein C, Khalil-Daher I, Dausset J, Carosella ED. Implication of HLA-G Molecule in Heart-Graft Acceptance. Lancet (London England) 2000; 355(9221): 2138. DOI: 10.1016/S0140-6736(00) 02386-2

[50] Lozano JM, González R, Kindelán JM, Rouas-Freiss N, Caballos R, Dausset J, et al. Monocytes and T Lymphocytes in HIV-1-Positive Patients Express HLA-G Molecule. AIDS (London England) 2002; 16(3): 347-351. DOI: 10.1097/00002030-200202150-00005

[51] Torres MI, Le Discorde M, Lorite P, Ríos A, Gassull MA, Gil A, et al. Expression of HLA-G in inflammatory bowel disease provides a potential way to distinguish between ulcerative colitis and Crohn's disease. Int Immunol. 2004; 16(4):579-83. DOI: 10.1093/intimm/dxh061.

[52] Shiroishi M, Tsumoto K, Amano K, Shirakihara Y, Colonna M, Braud V, et al. Human inhibitory receptors Ig-like transcript 2 (ILT2) and ILT4 compete with CD8 for MHC class I binding and bind preferentially to HLA-G. Proc Natl Acad Sci U S A. 2003; 100(15): 8856-8861. DOI: 10.1073/pnas.1431057100

[53] Anderson KJ, Allen R. Regulation of T-cell immunity by leucocyte immunoglobulin-like receptors: innate immune receptors for self on antigen-presenting cells. Immunology. 2009; 127(1): 8-17. DOI: 10.1111/j.1365-2567.2009. 03097.x

[54] Veit TD, Cordero EA, Mucenic T, Monticielo OA, Brenol JC, Xavier RM, et al. Association of the HLA-G 14bp polymorphism with systemic lupus erythematosus. Lupus 2009; 18: 424-30. DOI: 10.1177/0961203308098187

[55] Cordero EA, Veit TD, da Silva MA, Jacques SM, Silla LM, Chies JA. HLA-G polymorphism influences the susceptibility to HCV infection in sickle cell disease patients. Tissue Antigens 2009; 74: 308-13. DOI: 10.1111/j.1399-0039.2009 .01331.x

[56] Glas J, Torok HP, Tonenchi L, Wetzke M, Beynon V, Teshome MY, et al. The 14bp deletion polymorphism in the HLA-G gene display significant difference between ulcerative colitis and Crohn's disease and is associated with ileocecal resection in Crohn'disease. Int Immunol 2007; 16: 621-626. DOI: 10.1093/intimm /dxm027

[57] Rouas-Freiss N, Goncalves RM, Menier C, Dausset J, Carosella ED. Direct evidence to support the role of HLA-G in protecting the fetus from maternal uterine natural killer cytolysis. Proc Natl Acad Sci U S A 1997; 94: 11520-11525. DOI: 10.1073/pnas.94.21.11520

[58] LeMaoult J, Caumartin J, Daouya M, Favier B, Le Rond S, Gonzalez A, et al. Immune regulation by pretenders: cell-to-cell transfers of HLA-G make effector T cells act as regulatory cells. Blood 2007; 109: 2040-2048. DOI: 10.1182/blood-2006-05-024547

[59] Horuzsko A, Lenfant F, Munn DH, Mellor AL. Maturation of antigen presenting cells is compromised in HLA-G transgenic mice. Int Immunol 2001; 13: 385-394. DOI: 10.1093/intimm/13.3.385

[60] Carosella ED, HoWangYin KY, Favier B, LeMaoult J. HLA-G dependent suppressor cells: diverse by nature, function, and significance. Hum Immunol 2008; 69: 700-707. DOI: 10.1016/j.humimm.2008.08.280

[61] Torres MI, López-Casado MA, Luque J, Peña J, Ríos A. New advances in coeliac disease: serum and intestinal expression of HLA-G. *International Immunology*, 2006; 18 (5): 713-718. DOI: 10.1093/intimm/dxl008

[62] Torres MI, Lopez Casado MA, Rios A. New aspects in celiac disease. World J Gastroenterol 2007; 13: 1156-1161. DOI: 10.3748/wjg.v13.i8.1156

[63] Fabris A, Segat L, Catamo E, Morgutti M, Vendramin A, Crovella S. HLA-G 14bp deletion/insertion polymorphism in celiac disease. Am J Gastroenterol 2011; 106: 139-144. DOI: 10.1038/ajg.2010.340

[64] Catamo E, Zupin, Segat L, Celsi F, Crovella S. HLA-G and susceptibility to develop celiac disease. Human Immunology 2015; 76: 36-41. DOI: 10.1016/ j.humimm. 2014. 12.006

[65] Larsen MH, Hviid TV. Human leukocyte antigen-G polymorphism in relation to expression, function, and disease. Hum Immunol 2009; 70: 1026-1034. DOI: 10.1016/j.humimm.2009.07.015

[66] LeMaoult J, Krawice-Radanne I, Dausset J, Carosella ED. HLA-G1-expressing antigen-presenting cells induce immunosuppressive CD4+ T cells. Proc Natl Acad Sci USA 2004; 101: 7064-7069. DOI: 10.1073/pnas.0401922101

[67] Fournel S, Aguerre-Girr M, Huc X, Lenfant F, Alam A, Toubert A, et al. Cutting edge: soluble HLA-G1 triggers CD95/CD95 ligand-mediated apoptosis in activated CD8+ cells by interacting with CD8. J Immunol 2000; 164: 6100-6104. DOI: 10.4049/jimmunol.164.12.6100

[68] Donadi EA, Castelli EC, Arnaiz-Villena A, Roger M, Rey D, Moreau P. Implications of the polymorphism of HLA-G on its functions, regulation, evolution and disease association. Cell Mol Life Sci 2011; 68: 369-395. DOI: 10.1007/s00018-010-0580-7

[69] López AS, Alegre E, LeMaoult J, Carosella E, Gonzalez A. Regulatory role of tryptophan degradation pathway in HLA-G expression by human monocyte-derived dendritic cells. Mol Immunol. 2006; 43: 2151-2160. DOI: 10.1016/ j.molimm.2006.01.007

[70] Honing A, Rieger L, Kapp M, Sutterlin M, Dietl J, Kammerer U. Indoleamine 2, 3-dioxygenase (IDO) expression in invasive extravillous trophoblast supports role of the enzyme for maternal-tolerance. J Reprod Immunol. 2004; 61: 79-86. DOI: 10.1016/j.jri.2003.11.002

[71] Uyttenhove C, Pilotte L, Theate I, Stroobant V, Colau D, Parmentier N, et al. Evidence for a tumoral immune resistance mechanism based on tryptophan degradation by indoleamine 2,3-dioxygenase. Nat Med. 2003; 9: 1269-1274. DOI: 10.1038/nm934

[72] Takikawa O, Kuroiwa T, Yamazaki F, Kido R. Mechanism of interferon-gamma action. Characterization of indoleamine 2, 3-dioxygenase in cultured human cell induced by interferon-gamma and evaluation of the enzyme-mediated tryptophan degradation in its anticellular activity. J Biol Chem. 1998; 263: 2041-2048.

[73] Yang Y, Chu W, Geraghty D, Hunt J. Expression of HLA-G in human mononuclear phagocytes and selective induction of IFN-gamma. J Immunol. 1996; 156: 4224-4231.

[74] Moreau P, Adrian-Cabestre F, Menier C, Guiard V, Gourand L, Dausset J, et al. IL-10 selectively induces HLA-G expression in human trophoblast and monocytes. Int Immunol. 1999; 11: 803-811. DOI: 10.1093/ intimm/11.5.803

[75] González-Hernandez A, LeMaoult J, Lopez A, Alegre E, Caumartin, Le Rond S, Daouya. Linking Two Immuno-Suppressive Molecules: Indoleamine 2,3 Dioxygenase Can Modify HLA-G Cell-Surface Expression. Biol Reprod 2005; 73 (3):571-578, DOI: 10.1095/biolreprod.105.040089

[76] Fife BT, Bluestone JA. Control of peripheral T-cell tolerance and autoimmunity via the CTLA-4 and PD-1 pathways. Immunol Rev 2008; 224: 166-82. DOI: 10.1111/j.1600-065X.2008 .00662.x

[77] Simone R, Brizzolara R, Chiappori A, Milintenda-Floriani F, Natale C, Greco L, et al. A functional soluble form of CTLA-4 is present in the serum of celiac patients and correlates with mucosal injury. International Immunology, 2009; 21 (9): 1037-1045. DOI: 10.1093/intimm /dxp069

[78] Oaks MK, Hallett KM, Penwell R, Stauber EC, Warren SJ, Tector AJ. A native soluble form of CTLA-4. Cell Immunol. 2000; 201:144-153. DOI: 10.1006 /cimm. 2000.1649

[79] Brophy, K., Ryan, A. W., Thornton, J. M. Abuzakouk M, Fitzgerald AP, McLoughlin RM et al. Haplotypes in the CTLA4 region are associated with coeliac disease in the Irish population. Gen Immun. 2006; 7:19. DOI: 10.1038/ sj.gene .6364265

[80] Francisco LM, Sage PT, Sharpe AH. The PD-1 Pathway in Tolerance and Autoimmunity. Immunol Rev. 2010; 236: 219-242. DOI: 10.1111/j.1600065 X.2010. 00923.x

[81] Keir ME, Butte MJ, Freeman GJ, Sharpe AH. PD-1 and its ligands in tolerance and immunity. Annu Rev Immunol. 2008; 26: 677-704. DOI: 10.1146/annurev. immunol.26.021607.090331

[82] Agata Y, Kawasaki A, Nishimura H, Ishida Y, Tsubata T, Yagita H, Honjo T. Expression of the PD-1 antigen on the surface of stimulated mouse T and B lymphocytes. Int Immunol. 1996; 8: 765-772. DOI: 10.1093/intimm/8.5.765

[83] Kinter AL, Godbout EJ, McNally JP, Sereti I, Roby GA, O'Shea MA, Fauci AS. The common gamma-chain cytokines IL-2, IL-7, IL-15, and IL-21 induce the expression of programmed death-1 and its ligands. J Immunol. 2008; 181: 6738-6746. DOI: 10.4049/ jimmunol.181.10.6738

[84] Gianchecchi E, Fierabracci A. Inhibitory Receptors and Pathways of Lymphocytes: The Role of PD-1 in Treg Development and Their Involvement in Autoimmunity Onset and Cancer Progression. Front Immunol. 2018; 9: 2374. DOI: 10.3389/fimmu.2018.02374

[85] Sharpe AH, Pauken KE. The diverse functions of the PD1 inhibitory pathway. Nat Rev Immunol. 2018; 18(3): 153-167. DOI: 10.1038/nri.2017.108.

[86] Dezutter-Dambuyant C, Durand I, Alberti L, Bendriss-Vermare N, Valladeau-Guilemond J, Duc A. A novel regulation of PD-1 ligands on mesenchymal stromal cells through MMP-mediated proteolytic cleavage. Oncoimmunology. 2016; 5(3): e1091146. doi: 10.1080/ 2162402X. 2015.1091146

[87] Prokunina L, Castillejo-Lopez C, Oberg F, Gunnarsson I, Berg L,

Magnusson V, et al. A regulatory polymorphism in PDCD1 is associated with susceptibility to systemic lupus erythematosus in humans. Nat Genet. 2002; 32: 666-669. DOI: 10.1038/ng1020

[88] Liu C, Jiang J, Gao L, Hu X, Wang F, Shen Y, et al. A promoter region polymorphism in PDCD-1 gene is associated with risk of rheumatoid arthritis in the Han Chinese population of southeastern China. Int J Genomics. 2014; 2014: 247637. DOI: 10.1155/2014/247637

[89] Bertsias GK, Nakou M, Choulaki C, Raptopoulou A, Papadimitraki E, Goulielmos G et al. Genetic, immunologic, and immunohisto-chemical analysis of the programmed death 1/programmed death ligand 1 pathway in human systemic lupus erythematosus. Arthritis Rheum. 2009, 60(1): 207-218. DOI: 10.1002 /art.24227.

[90] Ponce de León C, López-Casado MA, Lorite P, Palomeque T, Torres MI. Dysregulation of the PD-1/PD-L1 pathway contributes to the pathogenesis of celiac disease. Cell Mol Immunol 2019; 16(9): 777-779. DOI: 10.1038/s41423-019-0256-7

[91] Abiko K, Matsumura N, Hamanishi J, Horikawa N, Murakami R, Yamaguchi K et al. IFN-γ from lymphocytes induces PD-L1 expression and promotes progression of ovarian cancer. Br J Cancer. 2015; 112(9): 1501-1509. DOI: 10.1038/bjc.2015.101

[92] Wu H, Miao M, Zhang G, Hu Y, Ming Z, Zhang X. Soluble PD-1 is associated with aberrant regulation of T cells activation in aplastic anemia. Immunol Invest. 2009;38:408-421. DOI: 10.1080/08820130902912332

[93] Carosella ED, Rouas-Freiss N, Tronik-Le Roux D, Moreau P, LeMaoult J. HLA-G: an immune checkpoint molecule. Adv Immunol. 2015; 1 27: 33-144. DOI: 10.1016/bs.ai.2015.04.001

[94] Zhang YH, Sun HX. Immune checkpoint molecules in pregnancy: Focus on regulatory T cells. Eur J Immunol. 2020; 50(2):160-169. DOI: 10.1002 /eji. 201948382

Chapter 4

Management of Patients with Refractory Coeliac Disease

Paul J. Ciclitira and Alastair Forbes

Abstract

Coeliac disease (CD) is an immune-mediated disorder affecting the small intestine. The condition represents an intolerance to gluten. Removal of dietary gluten permits recovery, with a full recovery for the majority of affected subjects. A percentage of affected subjects who do not improve with a gluten-free diet are considered to have refractory coeliac disease (RCD). Refractory coeliac disease is subdivided into type 1, characterised by a polyclonal expansion of intraepithelial lymphocytes (IELs) that have a normal phenotype, and type 2 (RCD2) which exhibits IELs with a monoclonal phenotype. Subjects with RCD carry a high risk of complications, including ulcerative jejunitis and lymphoma affecting the small intestine, the latter termed enteropathy-associated T-cell lymphoma (EATL).

Keywords: coeliac disease, refractory coeliac disease, presentation, diagnosis and treatment

1. Introduction

Coeliac disease (CD) represents an enteropathy affecting the small intestine that is exacerbated by gluten in wheat, rye and barley. The condition occurs in genetically susceptible individuals who carry either the HLA DQ2 or DQ8 genotype. [1] The prevalence of the condition, of which there is increasing awareness, is 1–2% in the US and Northern Europe. [2, 3]. Treatment of the condition comprises a gluten-free approach that involves removal of wheat, rye and barley from the diet. However, between 5 and 30% of affected subjects do not fully respond to a gluten-free diet, [2–6] and are considered to have refractory coeliac disease (RCD).

The precise diagnosis of RCD presents challenges, but is important in the development of new therapeutic strategies. [7–9]

2. Pathogenesis of RCD

Gluten proteins from wheat, rye and barley are divided into different groups. Wheat gluten comprises gliadin and glutenin. There are α, β, γ and ω gliadin fractions, and glutenin is composed of low and high molecular weight glutenins (HMWG). All these components of wheat gluten have been shown to be toxic to subjects with CD. [9]

In CD there is increased permeability of the small intestine associated with an increase in zonulin, a protein found between enterocytes that has been reported to be a modulator of tight junction permeability. [10, 11] It has been hypothesised that zonulin release induces increased absorption, into the lamina propria below the epithelium, of CD-toxic gluten fractions. The resultant gluten peptides in the lamina propria "stimulate aberrant adaptive and innate responses resulting in damage to the enterocytes, with infiltration of the mucosa by both intra-epithelial lymphocytes (IELs) and CD4 +ve lamina propria lymphocytes". Most of the increased number of IELs are CD3 + ve/CD8 + ve cells that express the α/β T-cell receptor (TCR), and a minority are γ/δ +ve (TCR)-expressing lymphocytes.

The adaptive response involves binding of the CD toxic peptides to HLA-DQ2 or HLA-DQ8. These reactive CD4 T-cells in the lamina propria recognise toxic gluten peptides and proteins. [12, 13] There is recognition of the gluten peptides bound to HLA-DQ2/DQ3, and to antigen presenting cells (APCs); this is enhanced by the enzyme tissue transglutaminase (tTg) that deamidates glutamine residues to glutamic acid [12]. Following activation of the T-cells, pro-inflammatory cytokines, including interferon-γ, are released. This in turn results in an inflammatory cascade, particularly affecting the proximal small intestine, that causes the observed villous atrophy [13].

The innate immune response appears to be mediated by IELs, enterocytes and dendritic cells, and is centred on increased secretion of the cytokine interleukin-15 (IL–15) [14]. It is possible that IL-15 production by enterocytes and dendritic cells is induced directly by gluten peptides. IL-15 stimulates the expression of MICA (a stress molecule) on enterocytes, and NKG2D (a natural killer receptor) on IELs. The IEL-induced NKG2D expression serves as an activating receptor with many ligands, including MICA [15]. In combination there may then be substantial cytotoxicity to enterocytes and thus the intestinal damage that is typical of CD.

It seems likely that RCD and uncomplicated CD have similar aetiopathogenic pathways. [14, 16] Most patients with RCD have increased levels of antigliadin and endomysial antibodies, although in RCD2 coeliac serology may become negative. Differentiation between RCD1 and RCD2 is based on evidence of either the polyclonal expansion of T-cells expression that occurs in RCD1, or the monoclonal expansion of T-cells in small intestinal biopsies or separated T-lymphocytes that can be demonstrated using double CD3/CD8 immuno-histochemistry in RCD2. An investigation of T-cell receptor clonal arrangements can be investigated by polymerase chain reaction on fresh tissue or by flow cytometry. [17–20]

The mechanisms behind the clonal expansion of T-cells in RCD2 are not well understood but there are several possibilities under active consideration. Genetic variation in the myosin IXB gene (MY09B) located on chromosome 19, has been proposed as a possible aetiopathological factor. [21] There is increased repairing of MICA and c-myc by the enterocytes [21–26]. An increase in IgM, Charcot-Leyden crystal proteins and apolipoprotein are observed and thought to be damaging in RCD2. [25] APO C3 apolipoprotein is also known to affect immunosurveillance cells, such as natural killer (NK) cells, and was singled out as potentially important in sustaining T-cell proliferation. [27]

IL-15 is overexpressed in untreated CD, and it is thought to play a pivotal role in the regulation of the IELs that characterise the disease and hence in in the pathogenesis of RCD. IELs show increased expression of IL-15Rα, elevated proliferation cytokine production and a reduction in apoptosis. [19]. It has been suggested also that IL-15 may induce the emergence of a clonal expression [19]. This multistep transformation may generate the pre-lymphomatous state and then progress to overt T-cell lymphoma [27]. Inhibition of IL-15 may have therapeutic value in RCD2 (see below) adding further weight to its suspected pathogenic importance.

3. Clinical features of RCD

3.1 Type 1 refractory coeliac disease

Patients with RCD1 may present with any combination of steatorrhoea, altered bowel habit (with both constipation and diarrhoea), abdominal pain, nausea, fatigue and weight loss [28]. RCD1 is also associated with thromboembolic infectious complications and autoimmune diseases. The radiological features on CT or MR scanning are similar to those of untreated CD, with increased ileal folds and decreased jejunal folds [29].

Patients with RCD1 exhibit Marsh type II or III appearances. [30] Both of these pathological gradings include villous atrophy. There is a moderate lymphoplasmacytic infiltrate in the lamina propria. [26] Collagen deposition (collagenous sprue) has been reported in 40% of patients with RCD1 [31]; this can be confirmed with a trichrome stain. Mucosal thinning with villous atrophy and crypt hyperplasia was reported in 30% of these patients.

The RCD1 IEL phenotype is equivalent to uncomplicated CD, with the majority of cells expressing CD3, CD7, CD8, CD103, and TCRβ. TCR gene rearrangement studies confirm that RCD1 cells constitute a polyclonal population. [28–32]

3.2 Type 2 refractory coeliac disease

RCD2 patients present with similar symptoms to those with RCD1, including malabsorption, weight loss, abdominal pain and diarrhoea. Most patients are aged 50–60. [28] The CT/MR appearances are similar to those in RCD1, but frequently also include lymphadenopathy, intussusception and hyposplenism. [29]

The standard histology of RCD2 mirrors RCD1, with the majority of patients demonstrating a degree of villous atrophy [30]. The cytological appearances of the IELs are normal. Cellier et al. [14] proposed that RCD2 (their refractory sprue) was associated with an abnormal subset of IELs that, on frozen section, were positive for CD103, CD7, and cytoplasmic CD3, but not for surface CD3, CD4, CD8, or TCRβ. This difference from RCD1 has contributed to the concept that RCD2 represents an early stage in the development of lymphoma. Aberrant IELs may also be found in gastric and colonic mucosa, and in the blood of RCD2 patients, implying that this is a diffuse gastrointestinal disease. The IELs in RCD2 patients rarely exhibit a normal CD3 + ve, CD8 + ve phenotype, and the majority have a CD3 + ve CD8 -ve pattern. However Goerres et al. [22] reported only a low frequency of loss of CD8 expression, and it is advocated that flow cytometry should be used to diagnose the condition.

Although a polyclonal IEL population has been reported in a very small proportion of RCD2 cases, it is usual to find monoclonality with a restricted rearrangement of the TCRβ gene when clonality studies are performed in RCD2.

4. Complications of RCD

4.1 Ulcerative Jejunitis

Most cases of ulcerative jejunitis (UJ) are preceded by problematic CD, such that UJ can be said to evolve from RCD. The mean age at onset of UJ is 50 years. The defining features are ulcerative lesions that are usually multifocal and which can involve the ileum as well as the jejunum. Presenting features include diarrhoea, steatorrhoea, abdominal pain and weight loss. There may be low grade fever, clubbing and nutritional deficiencies.

Mills et al. reported that the ulceration can extend through the full thickness of the mucosa, with secondary vascular changes [31] as well as submucosal oedema. There may also be fibrosis, leading to stricture formation. Complications can thus include haemorrhage, perforation and obstruction.

In some patients there is gastric metaplasia, and it is postulated that this contributes to ulcer formation. Most IELs in UJ have a phenotype identical to that of RCD2. The ulcers tend to show a mixed CD4 + ve/CD8 + ve and CD4-ve/CD8-ve phenotype. T-cell rearrangement studies identify clonality in the ulcers, the adjacent mucosa, or in both.

4.2 Enteropathy-type T-cell lymphoma

There is an increased risk of B- and T-cell lymphoma in coeliac disease. Enteropathy-associated T-cell lymphoma (EATL) is particularly linked to CD [29]. EATL usually presents with abdominal pain or overt intestinal perforation in adults with a background of RCD2 or UJ [33]. The strong association of EATL with HLA-DQB1 strengthens the inferred causal linkage between CD and EATL [33–36].

There are two main histological types of EATL. Type 1 is characterised by an infiltrate of medium sized cells containing round or angular nuclei with prominent nucleoli and a moderate amount of eosinophilic cytoplasm [33]. There may be marked pleomorphism with appearances like those of large-cell lymphoma or Hodgkin's lymphoma. The second, rarer type of EATL exhibits a monomorphic population of small, densely staining cells with hyperchromatic nuclei and minimal cytoplasm.

The malignant cells of both forms of EATL demonstrate monoclonality, with the same TCRγ gene rearrangement as seen in IELs in intestinal mucosa affected by the CD but which is uninvolved in the malignancy.

4.3 Other types of lymphoma

In addition to EATL, other types of non-Hodgkin's lymphoma are over-represented in patients with CD. Subtypes observed include B-cell neoplasms, follicular lymphoma, extranodal marginal zone lymphoma, and T-cell neoplasms.

4.4 Carcinoma of the GI tract

CD has an association with small bowel adenocarcinoma, which usually presents after the age of 45, with abdominal pain, weight loss, and/or anaemia. There is also an increased risk of squamous cell carcinoma of the upper digestive tract, including the oesophagus and oropharynx. There are minimally increased risks of primary liver cancer and of colorectal cancer.

5. Diagnostic approach to RCD

There are many reasons for patients with CD to fail to respond to a gluten-free diet, of which an underlying diagnosis of RCD is only one. [34] Poor dietary compliance and potential confusion of CD with other conditions should be excluded.

It has been suggested that a minimum of three properly orientated crypt to villous units are necessary for reliable interpretation of villous atrophy [34]. Helicobacter pylori, giardia, tuberculosis, tropical sprue, Whipple's disease, viral enteritis, AIDS, autoimmune enteritis, food protein intolerance, Crohn's disease, common variable immunodeficiency, collagenous sprue and eosinophilic gastroenteritis may all mimic CD [34]. Their exclusion from the differential diagnosis is not always straightforward when histological criteria are ambivalent or when multiple conditions co-exist (eg CD and infection).

The diagnosis of RCD runs in parallel with that of an initial comprehensive diagnosis of CD, which will therefore be briefly reprised. Coeliac serology should be obtained, with IgA and IgG antibodies to tissue transglutaminase and endomysium. Gliadin antibodies are unhelpful as IgG gliadin antibodies are raised in 5% of normal subjects, and in many of the conditions documented above, particularly Crohn's disease. HLA DQ2/DQ8 studies should be undertaken. A set of intestinal biopsies should be obtained for histological assessment. These endoscopic biopsies should be repeated after 4–6 months to confirm the diagnosis, and when RCD is suspected. [15]

In addition to evidence of villous atrophy, the biopsies will be examined for increased intraepithelial lymphocytes. The suggested normal upper limit for the small intestinal mucosa is 25 IELs per 100 enterocytes, with 25–29 considered borderline, and ≥ 30 IELs regarded as pathological lymphocytosis. In the normal small intestine there is a gradual reduction in the density of IELs between the bases and tips of the villi [37, 38]; a more even distribution of IELs along the lengths of the villi is strongly suggestive of underlying active CD [38, 39]. There is however a wide range of other conditions which cause intra-epithelial lymphocytosis, including *H. pylori* infection, enteric infarction, and autoimmune disease, and this may also occur with non-steroidal anti-inflammatory or other drugs.

According to the ESPGHAN diagnostic algorithm, the combination of a typical history, HLA-DQ2/8 positivity and coeliac serology at >10 x normal levels constitutes a diagnosis of coeliac disease in children [35]. Consequent to the COVID pandemic, the same diagnostic algorithm is now proposed for adults with symptoms of CD so long as they are ≤55 years of age, have no red flag symptoms, have a normal total IgA level, have an IgA tTG ≥ 10 times upper limit of normal, and a second positive antibody test such as anti-endomysial antibodies. However, most gastroenterologists feel this approach should only be temporary, as there is frequently discrepancy between the results of serology and small intestinal morphology [36, 40].

RCD will be considered in the patient who remains symptomatic or with persistently abnormal laboratory markers after apparent compliance with a gluten-free diet. Clinico-pathological correlation should first be undertaken to ensure that the initial diagnosis of CD was fully supported, including HLA DQ2/8 status, anti-endomysial and tissue transglutaminase antibodies, together with the presence of small bowel lesions, with particular attention to any history of a previous response to a gluten-free diet. RCD is however a histological diagnosis. Histological assessment will be particularly important where the initial diagnosis was made without a biopsy.

Appraisal of the gluten-free diet is crucial when contemplating RCD, as gluten contamination is the commonest cause of failure to respond to a gluten free diet. Contamination can be asymptomatic with minimal quantities, and can occur in patients who have received poor advice or are unaware of the broad range of products that can contain gluten [28].

In the absence of an aberrant IEL immunophenotype, the main differential diagnosis of CD-like histological lesions is limited to uncomplicated but inadequately treated CD, and RCD1. If there was no prior histology giving a diagnosis of CD, then a history of a previous response to a gluten-free diet is naturally highly supportive [28–36]. Both CD and RCD1 exhibit a polyclonal increase in IELs, mostly a CD3 + ve/CD8 + ve IEL population. Persistence or recurrence of small bowel lesions of this type, despite strict adherence to a gluten-free diet for at least one year, fulfils most observers' criteria for a diagnosis of RCD1.

The demonstration of a predominant CD3 + ve/CD8-ve aberrant IEL pheno-type leads to the consideration of RCD2 and its complications, including EATL. Polymerase chain reaction assessment of IELs and flow cytometry are now widely used to complement immunohistochemistry in the diagnosis of RCD2. These studies illustrate the importance of immune regulation in the likely pathogenesis of RCD and of RCD2 in particular.

Focal neoplasia (EATL and other forms) may be difficult to identify within the diffusely abnormal small intestine found in RCD2. Video capsule endoscopy, and PET-CT tomography scanning have been shown to be more effective in pinpointing EATL than CT alone. Video capsule endoscopy and subsequent enteroscopy are par-ticularly useful in detecting the more subtle lesions that may be the only macroscopic evidence of an underlying lymphoma. Elwenspoel *et al* propose to undertake an assessment of the accuracy of all potential diagnostic routes for coeliac disease and its complications involving a systematic review, the results of which are awaited [41].

6. Treatment of RCD

6.1 RCD1

All RCD patients should be reviewed by an expert dietitian in order to help them maximise their ability to adhere to a strict gluten-free diet.

In RCD1 the addition of systemic steroids has proven useful in some patients. The anti-TNFα biologic infliximab has also been proposed for the treatment of resistant coeliac disease [42]. Subsequent proposals have suggested a regimen of prednisolone and azathioprine that led to histological and clinical improvement in the majority of RCD1 patients following treatment for one year [22]. Dosages need some personalisation, but a tapering schedule of prednisolone (from 40 mg/day to less than 10 mg) with azathioprine at 2 mg/kg seem appropriate for most patients.

Use of an elemental diet not only provided clinical and histological improve-ment, but also reduced epithelial expression of the cytokine IL-15.

The specific defect in permeability associated with zonulin excess appears to be improved on treatment with larazotide acetate. [11]

6.2 RCD2

Prednisolone/azathioprine has been found to be helpful in some patients with RCD2 [8, 22].

Chemotherapy agents, such as the anti T-cell nucleoside analogues including pentostatin and cladribine have also been used with some success. [43]

Recently, IAMG 714, a monoclonal antibody to IL-15, has been studied in a randomised, double-blind, placebo-controlled, parallel-group trial in patients with type 2 refractory coeliac disease [44, 45].

Stem cell transplantation has been proposed as a therapeutic option, but this invasive approach is not generally accepted.

Overt lymphoma will be treated on standard oncological criteria and will normally fall outside the responsibility of the gastroenterologist.

7. Conclusions

In conclusion, the diagnosis of RCD is not straightforward. This interpretation of the clinical picture may have been incorrect, and the original diagnosis should always be reviewed, incorporating a re-assessment of the histology of small intestinal biopsies. Assessment of the gluten-free diet and correlation with the results of serology should be undertaken. PCR evaluation of biopsies or separated lymphocytes can be used to differentiate between RCD1 and RCD2, the former resembling severe but uncomplicated CD, while the latter typically has monoclonality and potentially premalignant features.

Treatment options have included steroids, azathioprine, infliximab, cladribine, stem cell transplantation and humanised monoclonal antibody to IL-15, (IAMG 714). There is to date no established standard intervention.

Acknowledgements

Ms. Janet Schulz kindly typed the first draft of the manuscript.

Neither PJ Ciclitira nor A Forbes holds current grant funding to support generation of this manuscript and there are no other potential conflicts of interest to declare.

Acronyms and non-standard abbreviations

APC	Anti-Presenting Cells
APO	Apolipoprotein
CD	Coeliac Disease
CT	Computed Tomography
EATL	Enteropathy-associated T-cell lymphoma
IELs	Intraepithelial lymphocytes
(Ig)A and (Ig)G	Immunoglobulins
IL	Interleukin
iNK	Invariant natural killer cells
MR	Magnetic resonance
NHL	Non-Hodgkin's lymphoma
NK	Natural killer
RCD	Refractory coeliac disease
TCR	T-cell receptor
tTG	Tissue transglutaminase
UJ	Ulcerative jejunitis

Author details

Paul J. Ciclitira[1*] and Alastair Forbes[1,2]

1 Department of Medicine, Norwich Medical School, University of East Anglia, Norwich, UK

2 Institute of Internal Medicine, University of Tartu, Tartu, Estonia

*Address all correspondence to: pciclitira@btinternet.com

IntechOpen

References

[1] Green PHR, Cellier C. Celiac disease. N. Engl. J. Med. 2007: 357: 1731-1743.

[2] van Heel DA, West J. Recent advances in coeliac disease. Gut 2006: 55; 1037-1046.

[3] Ciclitira PJ, King AL, Fraiser JS. AGA technical review on celiac sprue. American Gastroenterological Association. Gastroenterology 2001: 120; 1526-1540.

[4] Cellier C, Cerf-Bensussan N. Treatment of clonal refractory celiac disease or cryptic intraepithelial lymphoma: a long road from bench to bedside. Clin. Gastroenterol. Hepatol. 2006: 4; 1320-1321.

[5] Koning F. Celiac disease: caught between a rock and a hard place. Gastroenterology 2005: 129; 1294-1301.

[6] McGough N, Cummings JH. Coeliac disease: a diverse clinical syndrome, caused by intolerance of wheat, barley and rye. Proc. Nutr. Soc. 2005; 64; 434-450.

[7] Woodward J: The management of refractory coeliac disease. Therapeutic Advances in Chronic Coeliac Disease 2013; 4(2): 77-90.

[8] Nasr IK, Nasr IM, Beyers C, Chang F, Donnelly S, Ciclitira PJ, Recognising and Managing Refractory Coeliac Disease: A Tertiary Centre Experience. Nutrients. 2015 Dec; 7(12): 9896-9907.

[9] Kelly CP, Bai JC, Liu E, Leffler DA. Advances in diagnosis and management of celiac disease. Gastroenterology. 2015; 148(6): 1175-1186.

[10] Clemente MG, De Virgillis S, Kung JS. et al. Early effects of gliadin on enterocyte intracellular signaling involved in intestinal barrier function. Gut 2003: 52; 218-223.

[11] Fasano A, Not T, Wang W, et al. Zonulin, a newly discovered modulator of intestinal permeability, and its expression in coeliac disease. Lancet 2000: 3S5; 1518-1519.

[12] Rostoin A, Murray JA, Kagnoff MF. American Gastroenterological Association (AGA) Institute technical review on the diagnosis and management of celiac disease. Gastroenterology 2006; 131; 1982-2002.

[13] Craig D, Robins G, Howdle PD. Advances in celiac disease. Curr. Opin. Gastroenterology 2007; 23; 142-148.

[14] Cellier C, Delabesse E, Helmer C, et al. Refractory sprue, coeliac disease and enteropathy-associated T-cell lymphoma. French Coeliac Disease Study Group. Lancet 2000; 356: 203-208.

[15] Ludvigsson JF, Bai JC, Biagi F, Card TR, Ciacci C, Ciclitira PJ, Green PHR, et al Diagnosis and management of adult coeliac disease: guidelines from the British Society of Gastroenterology. Authors of the BSG Coeliac Disease Guidelines Development Group. Gut 2014; 63: 1210-1228.

[16] Koning F, Schuppan D, Cerf-Bensussan N, Sollid LM. Pathomechanisms in celiac disease. Best Pract. Res. Clin. Gastroenterol. 2005; 19; 373-387.

[17] Al-Toma A, Goerres MS, Meijer JWR, Peña AS, Crusius JBA, Mulder CJJ. Human leukocyte antigen-DQ2 homozygosity and the development of refractory celiac disease and enteropathy-associated T-cell lymphoma. Clin Gastroenterol Hepatol. 2006; 4(3): 315-319.

[18] Brousse N, Meijer JW. Malignant complications of coeliac disease. Best

Pract. Res. Clin. Gastroenterol. 2005: 19: 401-412.

[19] Di Sabatino A, Ciccocioppo R. Cupelli F, et al. Epithelium derived interleukin 15 regulates intraepithelial lymphocyte Th1 cytokine production. cytotoxicity. and survival in coeliac disease. Gut 2006: 55; 469-477.

[20] Cellier C, Patey N, Mauvieux L, Jabri B, Delabesse E, Cervoni JP, et al. Abnormal intestinal intraepithelial lymphocytes in refractory sprue. Gastroenterology 1998: 114: 471-481.

[21] Wolters VM, Verbeek WHM, Zhernakova A, Onland-Moret C, Schreurs MWJ, Monsuur AJ, Verduijn W, Wijmenga C, Mulder CJJ. The MYO9B gene is a strong risk factor for developing refractory celiac disease. Clin Gastroenterol Hepatol. 2007; 5(12):1399-1405.

[22] Goerres MS, Meijer JWR, Wahab PJ, Kerckhaert JAM, Groenen PJTA, van Krieken JHJM, Mulder CJJ. Azathioprine and prednisone combination therapy in refractory coeliac disease. Aliment Pharmacol Ther 2003;18(5):487-494.

[23] Ho-Yen C, Chang F, van der Walt J, Mitchell T, Ciclitira PJ. Recent advances in Refractory coeliac disease: a review. Histopathology 2009. 54, 783-795.

[24] Catassi C, Bearzi I, Holmes GKT. Association of celiac disease and intestinal lymphomas and other cancers. Gastroenterology 2005; 128(4/1):79-86.

[25] De Re V, Simula MP, Caggiari L, Orzes N, Spina M, Da Ponte A, De Appollonia L, Dolcetti R, Canzonieri V, Cannizzaro R. Proteins specifically hyperexpressed in a coeliac disease patient with aberrant T cells. Clin.Exp. Immunol. 2007; 148 : 402-409.

[26] Ciclitira PJ, Macartney JC, Evans G. Expressions of c-myc in non-malignant, and pre-malignant gastrointestinal disorders. J. Pathology 1987, 51; 293-296.

[27] Bernardo D, van Hoogstraten IMW, Verbeek WHM, Peña AS. Decreased circulating INKT cell numbers in refractory coeliac disease. Clinical Immunology 2008; 126(2):172-179.

[28] Daum S, Cellier C, Mulder CJ. Refractory coeliac disease. Best Pract. Res. Clin. Gastroenterol. 2005. 19: 413-424.

[29] Verkarre V, Asnafi V, Lecomte T, Patey Mariaud-De Serre N. Refractory coeliac sprue is a diffuse gastrointestinal disease. Gut 2003; 52(2):205-211.

[30] Marsh MN. Gluten, major histocompatibility complex, and the small intestine. A molecular and immunobiologic approach to the spectrum of gluten sensitivity ('celiac sprue'). Gastroenterology 1992; 102(1):330-354.

[31] Mills PR, Brown IL, Watkinson C. Idiopathic chronic ulcerative enteritis. Report of five cases and review of the literature. QJMed 1980: 49: 133-149.

[32] Bagdi E, Diss T, Munson P, Isaacson P. Mucosal intra-epithelial lymphocytes in enteropathy-associated T-cell lymphoma, ulcerative jejunitis, and refractory celiac disease constitute a neoplastic population. Blood 1999; 94: 260-264.

[33] Rooney N, Dogan A. Gastrointestinal lymphoma. Curr. Diagn. Pathol. 2004: 10; 69-78.

[34] Abdulkarim A, Burgart LJ, See J, Murray JA. Etiology of nonresponsive celiac disease: results of a systematic approach. Am. J. Gastroenterol. 2002: 97: 2016-2021.

[35] ESPGHAN 2020. New guidelines for the diagnosis of paediatric coeliac disease. https://www.espghan.org/

knowledge-center/publications/
Clinical-Advice-Guides/2020_New_
Guidelines_for_the_Diagnosis_of_
Paediatric_Coeliac_Disease. (Accessed
22/12/20).

[36] Penny HA, Sanders DS, Gillett H,
Gillett P, Edwards CM. Progress in
the serology-based diagnosis and
management of adult coeliac disease.
Expert Rev Gastroenterol Hepatol 2020.
13: 1-8.

[37] Hayat M, Cairns A, Dixon MF,
O'Mahony S. Quantitation of
intraepithelial lymphocytes in human
duodenum: what is normal? J. Clin.
Pathol. 2002: 55; 393-394.

[38] Veress B, Franzen L,
Bodin L, Borch K. Duodenal
lntraepithelial lymphocyte-count
revisited. Scand.]. Gastroenterology.
2004: 39; 138-144.

[39] Goldstein NS, Underhill J.
Morphologic features suggestive of
gluten sensitivity in architecturally
normal duodenum biopsy specimens.
Am. J. Clin. Pathol. 2001: 116; 63-71.

[40] Goldstein NS. Proximal small-
bowel mucosa! villous intraepithelial
lymphocytes. Histopathology 2004: 44;
199-205.

[41] Elwenspoek MMC, Jackson J,
Dawson S, Everitt H, Gillett P, Hay AD,
et al. Accuracy of potential diagnostic
indicators for coeliac disease: a
systematic review protocol. BMJ Open
2020; 10 (10): e038994.

[42] Chaudhary R, Ghosh S. lnfliximab
in refractory coeliac disease. Eur.
J. Gastroentrol. Hepatol. 2005 : 17;
603-604.

[43] Al-Toma A, Goerres MS,
Meijer JWR, von Blomberg BME,
Wahab PJ, Kerckhaert JAM, Mulder CJJ.
Cladribine therapy in refractory celiac
disease with aberrant T-cells. Clin.

Gastroenterol. Hepatol. 2006; 4(11):
1322-1327.

[44] Cellier C, Bouma G, van Gils T,
Khater S, Malamut G, Crespo L, et
al. Safety and efficacy of AMG 714 in
patients with type 2 refractory coeliac
disease: a phase 2a, randomised, double-
blind, placebo-controlled, parallel-
group study. Lancet Gastroenterol
Hepatol 2019. 4(12): 960-970.

[45] Vicari AP, Schoepfer AM,
Meresse B, Goffin L, Léger O,
Josserand S, et al. Discovery and
characterization of a novel humanized
anti-IL-15 antibody and its relevance
for the treatment of refractory celiac
disease and eosinophilic esophagitis.
MAbs 2017; 9: 927-944.

Chapter 5

Celiac Disease Management through Gluten-Free Diets

Babatunde Olawoye, Oseni Kadiri,

Oladapo Fisoye Fagbohun and Timilehin David Oluwajuyitan

Abstract

In recent times, there had been an increase in the consumption of food products made from cereals other than wheat flour. This is partly due to the surge or rise in wheat importation thereby led to a high foreign exchange spending for countries with comparative disadvantage in the cultivation and production of wheat grain. Aside from this, there had been a major concern on the health challenges emanating as a result of the consumption of food made from wheat flour. This health challenge is called celiac disease; an immune-mediated disease arising from the inability of the consumer to ingest gluten-containing products. This book chapter intends to write on the management of celiac disease using gluten-free diets.

Keywords: immune-mediated disorder, gluten-free diets, celiac disease: human leukocyte antigen

1. Introduction

In the last decade, there had been a rapid change in the dietary lifestyle among the world populace owing to increased globalization, urbanization and rapid economic development [1]. The rapid changes had also resulted in a large number of people suffering from poor health conditions due to the food they consume. Owing to this, there had been an increase in people's awareness about the role in which foods play in the emergence of these diseases [2–4]. One of such diseases resulting from food consumption is celiac disease (CD). Celiac disease, an autoimmune disorder, triggers when a genetically pre-disposed person or individual is exposed to dietary gluten resulting in the inflammation or damage of the lining of the small intestine. Celiac disease had become a global health challenge in which its prevalence is approximately 1% of the total world population with variation among regions, age, and sex [5]. However, there had been an increase in the prevalence of celiac disease in the US; a reason which was unclear but attributed to environmental component of celiac disease such as changes in the pattern of feeding, quality of ingested gluten, the spectrum of gastrointestinal infestation as well as the colonization of the gut microbiota. Symptoms associated with individuals suffering from celiac disease include retardation of growth, malnutrition, anemia, diarrhea as well as fatigue [6]. Currently, the only proven remedy for the treatment of celiac disease is the strict elimination of gluten from diets.

Generally, gluten is the term used to describe the alcohol-soluble fraction of storage protein in grain wheat which made up of most diet in western countries [7]. The storage proteins include prolamins (glutenin and gliadins) found in wheat grain, secalin found in rye, hordeins found in barley and avenins found in oats. These storage proteins had been found to contain glutamine and proline residues which are resistant to digestion in the gastrointestinal tract and encourage the deaminization by tissue trans-glutaminase [8]. These proteins when ingested by a genetically susceptible person caused a toxic effect on the gastrointestinal mucosa. The proteins activate the response by cellular immune leading to the injury of the intestinal mucosa which ranges from villous atrophy to infiltration of the lymphocytes. Villous atrophy in human leukocyte antigen (HLA) pre-disposed patient resulted in malabsorption of micro and macronutrients such as fat-soluble vitamins (A, D, E, K), folate, B complex vitamin (Niacin, riboflavin and thiamine), calcium, and iron. To revolve the menace, individuals suffering from a celiac disease needs to strictly adhere to gluten-free diets.

Gluten-free (GF) diets/foods are defined by the U.S. Food and Drug Administration as a food completely devoid of gluten or does not contain a gluten-containing grain (wheat, barley, oat and rye), flours made from gluten-containing grain in which the gluten had been removed or not removed (wheat flour or starch) and finally, if any of the above-mentioned products contain at least 20 ppm of gluten in food [9]. However, the Commission Regulation of European Union defines a gluten-free diet as a foodstuff that contains a gluten level not exceeding 20 ppm for people who are intolerance to gluten. It was further regulated that food not exceeding 100 ppm in gluten content should be tagged as very low gluten. There is a wide range of palatable and attractive gluten-free diets specifically manufactured for individuals suffering from celiac disease and this include but not limited to GFD baked products, beverage drinks, wines, beers, sourdough etc. [10, 11]. These products are cereal-based food and had gained wide visibility in North and South America, Europe, North Africa and some part of Asia. Gluten-free products' marketability is estimated to increase in value from US$ 4.18 billion in 2017 to US$ 6.47 billion by 2023 in which gluten-free bread and cookie are estimated to be the most consumed cereal-based GF-food globally [9]. During the production of food products made from gluten, gluten present in the food products is responsible for the elasticity, extensivity and texture resistant if the dough [2, 12]. However, to improve the quality (texture and specific volume) of gluten-free diet/products, hydrocolloids such as hydroxypropylmethylcellulose, xanthan gum, pectin, carboxymethylcellulose are commonly used to improve the baking quality, imparting texture and appearance as well as stability in the gluten-free dough.

2. Nutritional properties of gluten-free diet

Though gluten-free products are ideal for consumption by patients living with the celiac disease, it is however low in protein due to the utilization of flour and starches with higher starch to protein content. When flours from pulses are blended with gluten-free cereals, it results in a meal with the complementary amino acid profiles and likewise provides high-quality proteins for bakery purposes. C-ertain species of pseudocereals have been reported to have significant nutritional constituents such as micronutrients, polyphenols, proteins, and dietary fibers when compared with flour produced from cereals [13]. Significant higher mineral content has been reported in gluten-free foods produced from quinoa, millet, oat, amaranth, and buckwheat when compared with those made from rice, maize, and potato starch [13].

Some method which had been reported to improve nutritional values and bioavailability of gluten-free bakery goods includes malting and sprouting as these processes help in activating enzymes responsible for the starch, proteins, and lipids breakdown [14, 15]. It has been suggested that gluten-free bakery products should be incorporated with pulses and pseudocereals rather than the use of starches and gluten-free cereals only.

2.1 Sensory properties of gluten-free diet

A major challenge in the production of gluten-free bakery products is in achieving sensory attributes that are desirable and acceptable by consumers. Gluten-free bakery products are known for their distinct color, texture, appearance, taste, and aroma when compared to those made from wheat flour. Due to complex formulation, gluten-free bakery products tend to appear darker. Regarding wheat products, gluten-free bakery products have lower volumes and harder textures. The acceptability of some gluten-free bakery products has been reported to improve in terms of texture when some proteins were added. In a study by Matos *et al.* [16], gluten-free muffins were more acceptable by consumers when soy protein isolate was incorporated. In a related study, the acceptability of millet muffins improved in terms of texture when chicken protein isolate and transglutaminase were combined [17]. Future research should focus on how enzymes, proteins, hydrocolloids, and other ingredients can improve the sensory acceptability of gluten-free bakery and pasta products.

2.2 Gluten-free products/diets used in managing celiac disease

A very good way of managing celiac disease in immune-mediated patients is the total exclusion of gluten from their diet and diet substitution using gluten-free products. The underlisted products are gluten-free products commonly used in the treatment and management of celiac disease.

2.2.1 GF-dough/sourdough

GF-dough is a thick, malleable mixture of flour (usually cereal - wheat, barley, and rye) and liquid (water) used in the production of bakery products void of gluten. Total removal of gluten from these products enhance safety consumption for celiac disease patients. However, this comes with several difficulties such as poor dough rheological properties, reduced nutritional qualities, off flavor, poor mouth-feel/taste, and more expensive GF-baked product compared with conventional gluten baked products [18–20].

In research for remedy, food products have been developed from GF-dough made from GF-flour (such as rice, sorghum, buckwheat, amaranth, quinoa, and maize) [19, 21], dairy products [22], dietary fibers [3, 23], and starches [2–4]. Advantages of these alternatives are low glycemic index, antihypertensive, and antihyperlipidemia [2–4].

Recently, researches have also focused on the production of food products from sourdough rather than from gluten flour [24–26]. Sourdough is described as a product of a biotechnological process that involves the mixture of flour (cereal) and water, fermented by lactic acid bacteria thereby causing a pleasant sour-tasting dough/product [27]. Sourdough is used to produce several varieties of baked products such as bread, biscuits (crackers) and cakes. Before production, sourdough is characterized by increase dough leavening which promotes GF-end product attractiveness, improved texture and palatability, increase mineral bioavailability, slow down the rate of starch digestion (low glycemic index), antihypertensive potential and extended shelf-life GF-products [19, 26, 28]. Sourdough applications also include the production of novel bioactive compounds which can be used as pre-bioactive starter cultures [28–30].

2.2.2 GF-baked products

Understanding the functionality of gluten is very important in the baking process of convectional product made from wheat. This gives an insight into the most suitable ingredients that can be considered as gluten replacement. Gluten-free bread has been produced from several types of gluten-free flour such as pseudocereals (e.g., Buckwheat, quinoa, amaranth) [31, 32], cereals (e.g., sorghum, maize, rice) [33, 34], and potato flour [35]. A gluten substitute in bread-making is hydrocolloid. Some commonly reported hydrocolloids include; hydroxypropylmethylcellulose [36]; xanthan gum [32], carboxymethylcellulose, and apple pectic [35]. The application of buckwheat in the production of gluten-free bakery products such as noodle, pasta, cookie, and bread has been reviewed by Giménez-Bastida *et al.* [37]. The sensory acceptability and present technological limitations of gluten-free pasta and bread were reviewed by Padalino *et al.* [4]. Strategies for enhancing the quality of gluten-free noodles, pasta, and bread were likewise reviewed by Collar [38], Elgeti *et al.* [39], and Naqash *et al.* [40]. Aside from the formulation of gluten-free baked products from cereals and pseudocereals, there had also been a report of the production of GF-baked products such as bread, pastries and cookies from starch isolated from root and tuber crops, banana, cereals and legumes [2–4, 12, 41].

2.2.3 Gluten-free noodles

A diet which is free of gluten is the most effective therapy for ailment such as celiac disease. Aside from its beneficial roles in patients with celiac disease, it also has some perceived health benefits such as the regulation weight loss regulation and prevention of gastrointestinal disease. The gluten-free industry was reported to experience a growth of 136% between 2013 and 2015 [42]. Aside from the conventional production of noodles from wheat, noodles are also produced from other uncommon sources such as starches derived from corn, cassava, potatoes, mung beans, and konjac. Grains of rice, oats, and buckwheat are other unconventional sources.

Several grain varieties were also used in the production of gluten-free noodles with good nutritional and health values. Gluten-free noodles are most suitable for consumption by patients with intolerance to gluten as found in patients with celiac disease. This type of noodles is mostly recommended for anyone who needs to avoid the health challenges posed by the consumption of gluten foods.

Noodles made from rice grains are the second most common products after cooked rice grains. Noodles are mostly produced from Indica rice variety and very common in Asia countries like the Philippines, Sri Lanka, Vietnam, Thailand, and Sri Lanka. Fu [43] classified rice noodles into instant, frozen, dried products of shapes and thickness of differing types. With an amylose content of over 22%, Indica rice is most suitable for noodles production. The starch properties determine the structural characteristics of rice noodles as its constituent protein does not play any role in the formation of a stable network structure [44].

Rice noodles are not prone to breaking apart when pan-fried. They also have an elastic and flexible texture when pan-fried. Majority of consumers preferred rice noodles which are boiled, pan-fried or soup with several ingredients as this noodle products have a smooth taste when eaten and improved eating qualities. Aside from its amylose which is viewed as a possible reason for its suitability in rice noodles production, the exact mechanism is not understood fully.

Oat grain is a herb plant grown annually. The consumer market for this plant is small. The two major types of oats are *Avena nuda* L. (naked oats) and *Avena sativa* L. (*Avena sativa*). *Avena nuda* L. is the most commonly cultivated oat in the

Gansu, Hebei, Jilin, and Inner Mongolia Provinces in China. Oats are highly nutritious, high-energy and low-sugar food. Oats are usually referred to as healthy foods because of their ability to regulate the metabolism of cholesterol, thereby impeding the onset of certain ailment such as cardiovascular disease, aside its other health benefits [45].

Buckwheat flour has protein content within the range of 7–13%, which is significantly higher than the values present in wheat and rice flour. Buckwheat flour is also rich in linoleic and oleic acid with a fat content of about 3%. Rutin, a bioactive compound with hypertensive and hypolipidemic effects, is present in buckwheat flour. Buckwheat noodles are majorly produced in northeast China, Korea, and Japan. Buckwheat noodles processing can be either slit buckwheat noodles or extruded buckwheat noodles. Just like in wheat noodles production, buckwheat noodles are also produced manually or mechanically. In studies by Alamprese et al. [46], pasta product was developed from a combination of eggs, rice flour, and buckwheat flour. This study demonstrates the potential of buckwheat use for noodles production without incorporating wheat flour which is gluten carrying constituent.

Cassava noodles, potato noodles, konjac noodles, corn noodles, mung bean noodles etc. are some other types of noodles product which are gluten-free. These noodles are rich in nutritional and functional values [47–51]. **Figure 1** shows the flowchart for noodle processing.

2.2.4 GF-beverage/functional drinks based on cereal

GF-beverage is another GF-product made from GF-cereals such as teff, millet, tigernut, acha, fonio, sorghum among others, consume for prevention/management of celiac disease. Some also play an additional role in the body beyond basic nutritional needs and served as functional drinks. Teff is GF-grain suitable for wheat/barley replacement in production of GF-beverage. Gebremariam et al. [52] reported on Ethiopia local functional drinks made from teff. It was observed that the GF-functional drink exhibits medicinal potential and is suitable for the management of malaria, anemia and diabetes. Badejo et al. [53] developed a GF-beverage from the combination of tigernut and acha varying the blending ratios at 25%. It was observed that the developed beverages contain an appreciable number of phenolic compounds such as gallic acid, rutin, quercetin, ellagic and caffeic acids which may be responsible for higher free radical scavenging abilities reported against DPPH* and ABTS*. Sharma et al. [54] developed prebiotic oligosaccharide rich GF-functional drink from sorghum. They highlighted that the GF-functional drink is suitable for celiac disease patient and contains high calories value, antioxidant capacity, and no changes in sensory properties compared with wheat/barley beverage. GF-beverage are relatively cheap and have extended shelf-life [55].

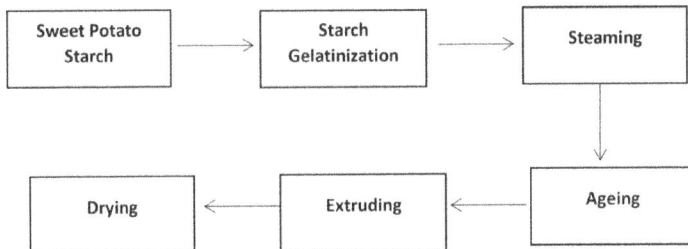

Figure 1.
Potato noodles processing flowchart.

2.2.5 Gluten-free beer

Beer is an alcoholic carbonated, and fermented beverage produced from malted cereal grain (such as wheat, barley, and rye). Consumption of beer is toxic to celiac patients and could results into this autoimmune disorder due to the presence of gliadin from wheat gluten, prolamines/hordeins from barley, and secalins from rye [19, 56]. Scientific research has shown that the successful long-term management of this autoimmune disorder is strict adherence to GF diets [57–59]. Hence, the needs for GF-beer. European Commission guidelines described GF-beer as pseudo-cereals/cereal malted beer devoid of gluten or beer technologically produced from brewing malt to reduced its gluten content to less than 20 mg/kg [60, 61]. However, controversy exists as US Food and Drug Administration (FDA) proclaim the latter product has the potential to exhibits celiac symptoms in some patients than the former [62, 63].

Pseudo-cereals malted beer produced from amaranth, buckwheat, and quinoa free of gluten is therefore recommended for celiac patient [56, 57, 64]. These malted beers contain adequate proteins and relatively high starch with sensory attributes slightly lower compared to beer produced from wheat and barley in respect to their taste, aroma, and mouthfeel when adequately mashed, fermented, and stabilized. However, the cost of technology to achieve the aforementioned may inflate the price of pseudo-cereal beer [56, 65].

Alternatively, GF-beer can also be produced from GF-cereal such as sorghum, rice, and maize with several brewing conditions been altered such as mashing, sparging, boiling, fermentation temperatures, and pH [66, 67]. This adjust-ment relatively increases their disparities compared with wheat and barley beer. Comparing GF-sorghum beer with barley beer, the former is rather too viscous, slightly sweetish, and a little bit sour due to the formation of lactic acid [68]. Ceppi and Brenna [69] observed that rice GF-beer were acceptable by consumers but had lower enzymatic activity than barley. Zweytik and Berghofer [68] also reported that GF-maize beer is light yellow with good foam stability, but was relatively poor in taste compared with barley beer. However, they tend to have higher demands by the consumers due to their cheap price [66].

3. Market feasibility of GF diets/foods

Owing to increase in patients suffering from celiac disease as well as gluten intolerance, there had been a rise in consumer demand for gluten-free products as a result of the increase in the number of diagnosis as well as consumers who are making a conscious choice or effort to exclude gluten from their diets. The demand had made gluten-free products one of the fastest-growing market opportunity within the consumer wellness and global health market. For a patient who requires a gluten-free diet, the products must be the same in terms of texture and appearance as conventional gluten-containing products. A market survey of gluten-free food in the United State of America (USA) reveals that the market stood at $2.3 billion in 2019 and it's estimated to reach $4.5 billion by 2027 according to Gorgitano and Sodano [70]. The United Kingdom (UK) gluten-free products, however, was estimated to be £426 million in 2018 and it's expected to grow by 40% by 2030. The estimated increase in gluten-free products in the US and UK was due to the facts that gluten-free products are alternative to conventional and traditional grain-based food products such as bakery, pastries, pasta-products which can be made alternatively from other cereals such as maize, sorghum, millet as well as rice [71]. Although the market of gluten-free products had surged higher than the products for other medically diagnosed gluten-related diseases, however, the demand is lower in comparison with gluten-containing products. This had been attributed to the perception of gluten-free products by the consumers as poor or lower quality products with poor appearance, flavor, and texture [1]. However, due to the adherence to gluten-free diets by patients suffering from celiac or gluten intolerance disease, there had been an additional economic burden on the patients due to higher cost price of the products when compared to conventional non-gluten-free products found in the market. In addition to the high selling price of the gluten-free diets, there had been a problem of its availability in the market [72]. A general survey on the market price of gluten-free foods over gluten-containing food products revealed that the price of gluten-free products was 242% more expensive than conventional gluten-containing products. The price was, however, found to be 89% more expensive than its regular products in Chile. The evaluation of the market price, availability and the nutritional composition of gluten-free products by Bagolin do Nascimento et al. [72] at the capital city of Brazil revealed the limitation in the availability of the products in the market coupled with high selling price in comparison with conventional products. Concerning market size among the different segment of gluten-free products, it was reported that gluten-free cookies had more sales and brought in more money compared to gluten-free bread, a reason which could be attributed to the convenience and the quality of the cookie [73]. Other reason could be the importance of gluten in the functional properties of the bread compared to cookie. Gluten gives desirable quality such as the loaf texture and volume to the bread. To make gluten-free foods or products available and avoidable to the patients, the price of the develop GF-foods needs to be considered.

4. Conclusion

An approximately 1% of the people living in the world today suffers from celiac disease. However, there had been an uprise in the prevalence of the disease due to the underestimation of the disease as it is often left undiagnosed. The only proven remedy to the treatment and management of the disease is the exclusion of wheat or gluten-containing products from their diet and through adherence to gluten-free products/foods. One constrains being perceived by patient suffering from celiac disease is the nutritional imbalance of the diets as a result of the exclusion of gluten and other major gluten-related protein from their diets. Owing to this, it is important that when developing gluten-free diets for patients suffering from celiac disease, the GF-food should be of high nutritional composition, available, and avoidable economically.

Author details

Babatunde Olawoye[1*], Oseni Kadiri[2], Oladapo Fisoye Fagbohun[3]
and Timilehin David Oluwajuyitan[4]

1 Department of Food Science and Technology, First Technical University, Ibadan,
Oyo State, Nigeria

2 Department of Biochemistry, Edo University Iyamho, Auchi, Edo State, Nigeria

3 Department of Biomedical Engineering, First Technical University, Ibadan,
Oyo State, Nigeria

4 Department of Food Science and Technology, Federal University of Technology
Akure, Nigeria

*Address all correspondence to: btolawoye@gmail.com

IntechOpen

References

[1] Jnawali, P., Kumar, V., & Tanwar, B. (2016). Celiac disease: Overview and considerations for development of gluten-free foods. Food Science and Human Wellness, 5(4), 169-176. https://doi.org/https://doi.org/10.1016/j.fshw.2016.09.003

[2] Olawoye, B., Gbadamosi, S. O., Otemuyiwa, I. O., & Akanbi, C. T. (2020a). Gluten-free cookies with low glycemic index and glycemic load: optimization of the process variables via response surface methodology and artificial neural network. Heliyon, 6(10), e05117. https://doi.org/https://doi.org/10.1016/j.heliyon.2020.e05117

[3] Oluwajuyitan, T. D., Ijarotimi, O. S., & Fagbemi, T. N. (2020). Nutritional, biochemical and organoleptic properties of high protein-fibre functional foods developed from plantain, defatted soybean, rice-bran and oat-bran flour. Nutrition & Food Science.

[4] Padalino, L., Conte, A., & Del Nobile, M. A. (2016). Overview on the general approaches to improve gluten-free pasta and bread. Foods, 5(4), 87.

[5] DeGeorge, K. C., Frye, J. W., Stein, K. M., Rollins, L. K., & McCarter, D. F. (2017). Celiac Disease and Gluten Sensitivity. Primary Care: Clinics in Office Practice, 44(4), 693-707. https://doi.org/10.1016/j.pop.2017.07.011

[6] Grace-Farfaglia, P. (2015). Bones of contention: bone mineral density recovery in celiac disease--a systematic review. Nutrients, 7(5), 3347-3369. https://doi.org/10.3390/nu7053347

[7] Schuppan, D., & Zimmer, K.-P. (2013). The diagnosis and treatment of celiac disease. Deutsches Arzteblatt international, 110(49), 835-846. https://doi.org/10.3238/arztebl.2013.0835

[8] Itzlinger, A., Branchi, F., Elli, L., & Schumann, M. (2018). Gluten-Free Diet in Celiac Disease-Forever and for All? Nutrients, 10(11). https://doi.org/10.3390/nu10111796

[9] Xu, J., Zhang, Y., Wang, W., & Li, Y. (2020). Advanced properties of gluten-free cookies, cakes, and crackers: A review. Trends in Food Science & Technology, 103, 200-213. https://doi.org/https://doi.org/10.1016/j.tifs.2020.07.017

[10] Tebben, L., Shen, Y., & Li, Y. (2018). Improvers and functional ingredients in whole wheat bread: A review of their effects on dough properties and bread quality. Trends in Food Science & Technology, 81, 10-24. https://doi.org/https://doi.org/10.1016/j.tifs.2018.08.015

[11] Xu, J., Wang, W., & Li, Y. (2019). Dough properties, bread quality, and associated interactions with added phenolic compounds: A review. Journal of Functional Foods, 52, 629-639. https://doi.org/https://doi.org/10.1016/j.jff.2018.11.052

[12] Olawoye, B., & Gbadamosi, S. O. (2020). Sensory profiling and mapping of gluten-free cookies made from blends Cardaba banana flour and starch. Journal of Food Processing and Preservation, 44(9), e14643. https://doi.org/10.1111/jfpp.14643

[13] Di Cairano, M., Galgano, F., Tolve, R., Caruso, M. C., & Condelli, N. (2018). Focus on gluten free biscuits: Ingredients and issues. Trends in Food Science & Technology, 81, 203-212.

[14] Eskin, M., & Shahidi, E. (2013). Biochemistry of foods. The Quarterly Review of Biology, 88 (2), 142.

[15] Miranda-Villa, P. P., Mufari, J. R., Bergesse, A. E., & Calandri, E. L. (2019). Effects of Whole and Malted Quinoa Flour Addition on Gluten-Free

Muffins Quality. Journal of food science, *84*(1), 147-153.

[16] Matos, M. E., Sanz, T., & Rosell, C. M. (2014). Establishing the function of proteins on the rheological and quality properties of rice based gluten free muffins. Food Hydrocolloids, *35*, 150-158.

[17] Shaabani, S., Yarmand, M. S., Kiani, H., & Emam-Djomeh, Z. (2018). The effect of chickpea protein isolate in combination with transglutaminase and xanthan on the physical and rheological characteristics of gluten free muffins and batter based on millet flour. LWT, *90*, 362-372.

[18] Arendt, E. K. (2002). *O, brien, CM, Schober, T. J., Gallagher, E. & Gormley* (pp. 21-27). TR.

[19] Arendt, E. K., Moroni, A., & Zannini, E. (2011). Medical nutrition therapy: use of sourdough lactic acid bacteria as a cell factory for delivering functional biomolecules and food ingredients in gluten free bread. In *Microbial Cell Factories* (Vol. 10, No. S1, p. S15). BioMed Central.

[20] Arendt, E. K., Morrissey, A., Moore, M. M., & Dal Bello, F. (2008). Application of dairy ingredients in gluten-free food. Gluten-Free Cereal Products and Beverages, 228-231.

[21] Cappelli, A., Oliva, N., & Cini, E. (2020). A Systematic Review of Gluten-Free Dough and Bread: Dough Rheology, Bread Characteristics, and Improvement Strategies. Applied Sciences, *10*(18), 6559.

[22] Graça, C., Mota, J., Lima, A., Boavida Ferreira, R., Raymundo, A., & Sousa, I. (2020). Glycemic Response and Bioactive Properties of Gluten-Free Bread with Yoghurt or Curd-Cheese Addition. Foods, *9*(10), 1410.

[23] Ijarotimi, O. S., Oluwajuyitan, T. D., & Ogunmola, G. T. (2019). Nutritional, functional and sensory properties of gluten-free composite flour produced from plantain (Musa AAB), tigernut tubers (Cyperus esculentus) and defatted soybean cake (Glycine max). Croatian journal of food science and technology, *11*(1), 1131-1251.

[24] Alibašić, H., Junuzović, H., Selimović, A., Selimović, A., & Brčina, T. (2020). Chemical Composition and Sensory Properties of Gluten-Free Crackers with Buckwheat Sourdough. International Journal for Research in Applied Sciences and Biotechnology, *7*(4), 108-113.

[25] Alioğlu, T., & Özülkü, G. (2020). Evaluation of whole wheat flour sourdough as a promising ingredient in short dough biscuits. Food Science and Technology, (AHEAD).

[26] Diowksz, A., Malik, A., Jaśniewska, A., & Leszczyńska, J. (2020). The Inhibition of Amylase and ACE Enzyme and the Reduction of Immunoreactivity of Sourdough Bread. Foods, 9(5), 656.

[27] Chavan, R. S., & Chavan, S. R. (2011). Sourdough technology—a traditional way for wholesome foods: a review. Comprehensive Reviews in Food Science and Food Safety, 10(3), 169-182.

[28] Katina, K., Arendt, E., Liukkonen, K. H., Autio, K., Flander, L., & Poutanen, K. (2005). Potential of sourdough for healthier cereal products. Trends in Food Science & Technology, 16(1-3), 104-112.

[29] Maidana, S. D., Ficoseco, C. A., Bassi, D., Cocconcelli, P. S., Puglisi, E., Savoy, G., ... & Fontana, C. (2020). Biodiversity and technological-functional potential of lactic acid bacteria isolated from spontaneously fermented chia sourdough. International journal of food microbiology, *316*, 108425.

[30] Olojede, A. O., Sanni, A. I., Banwo, K., & Adesulu-Dahunsi, A. T. (2020).

Sensory and antioxidant properties and in-vitro digestibility of gluten-free sourdough made with selected starter cultures. *LWT*, 109576.

[31] Burešová, I., Tokár, M., Mareček, J., Hřivna, L., Faměra, O., & Šottníková, V. (2017). The comparison of the effect of added amaranth, buckwheat, chickpea, corn, millet and quinoa flour on rice dough rheological characteristics, textural and sensory quality of bread. Journal of Cereal Science, *75*, 158-164.

[32] Hager, A. S., & Arendt, E. K. (2013). Influence of hydroxypropylmethylcellulose (HPMC), xanthan gum and their combination on loaf specific volume, crumb hardness and crumb grain characteristics of gluten-free breads based on rice, maize, teff and buckwheat. Food Hydrocolloids, *32*(1), 195-203.

[33] Monthe, O. C., Grosmaire, L., Nguimbou, R. M., Dahdouh, L., Ricci, J., Tran, T., & Ndjouenkeu, R. (2019). Rheological and textural properties of gluten-free doughs and breads based on fermented cassava, sweet potato and sorghum mixed flours. LWT, *101*, 575-582.

[34] Wu, T., Wang, L., Li, Y., Qian, H., Liu, L., Tong, L., ... & Zhou, S. (2019). Effect of milling methods on the properties of rice flour and gluten-free rice bread. LWT, *108*, 137-144.

[35] Liu, X., Mu, T., Sun, H., Zhang, M., Chen, J., & Fauconnier, M. L. (2018). Influence of different hydrocolloids on dough thermo-mechanical properties and in vitro starch digestibility of gluten-free steamed bread based on potato flour. Food Chemistry, *239*, 1064-1074.

[36] Mancebo, C. M., San Miguel, M. Á., Martínez, M. M., & Gómez, M. (2015). Optimisation of rheological properties of gluten-free doughs with HPMC, psyllium and different levels of water. Journal of cereal science, *61*, 8-15.

[37] Giménez-Bastida, J. A., Piskuła, M., & Zieliński, H. (2015). Recent advances in development of gluten-free buckwheat products. Trends in Food Science & Technology, *44*(1), 58-65.

[38] Collar, C. (2019). Gluten-free dough-based foods and technologies. In J. R. N. Taylor, & K. G. Duodu (Eds.), *Sorghum and millets: Chemistry, technology and nutritional attributes* (pp. 331-354). Published by Elsevier Inc. in cooperation with AACC International.

[39] Elgeti, D., Jekle, M., & Becker, T. (2015). Strategies for the aeration of gluten-free breads - a review. Trends in Food Science & Technology, *46*, 75-84.

[40] Naqash, F., Gani, A., Gani, A., & Massodi, F. A. (2017). Gluten-free baking: Combating the challenges - a review. Trends in Food Science & Technology, *66*, 98-107.

[41] Adiamo, O. Q., Fawale, O. S., & Olawoye, B. (2018). Recent Trends in the Formulation of Gluten-Free Sorghum Products. Journal of Culinary Science & Technology, *16*(4), 311-325. https://doi.org/10.1080/15428052.2017.1388896

[42] Gobbetti, M., Pontonio, E., Filannino, P., Rizzello, C. G., De Angelis, M., & Di Cagno, R. (2018). How to improve the gluten-free diet: The state of the art from a food science perspective. Food Research International, *110*, 22-32.

[43] Fu, B. X. (2008). Asian noodles: History, classification, raw materials, and processing. Food Research International, *41*(9), 888-902.

[44] Kim, Y., Kee, J. I., Lee, S., & Yoo, S. H. (2014). Quality improvement of rice noodle restructured with rice protein isolate and transglutaminase. Food Chemistry, *145*, 409-416.

[45] Tong, L. T., Guo, L., Zhou, X., Qiu, J., Liu, L., Zhong, K., & Zhou, S. (2016). Effects of dietary oat proteins on cholesterol metabolism of hypercholesterolaemic hamsters. Journal of the Science of Food and Agriculture, *96*(4), 1396-1401.

[46] Alamprese, C., Casiraghi, E., & Pagani, M. A. (2007). Development of gluten-free fresh egg pasta analogues containing buckwheat. European Food Research and Technology, *225*(2), 205-213.

[47] Akanbi, C. T., Kadiri, O., & Gbadamosi, S. O. (2019). Kinetics of starch digestion in native and modified sweet potato starches from an orange fleshed cultivar. International journal of biological macromolecules, *134*, 946-953.

[48] Gbadamosi, S. O., Kadiri, O., & Akanbi, C. T. (2020). Quality Characteristics of Noodles Produced from Soybean Protein Concentrate and Sweet Potato Starch: A Principal Component and Polynomial Cubic Regression Model Approach. *Journal of Culinary Science & Technology*, 1-21.

[49] Renaud, S., & Lanzmann-Petithory, D. (2001). Coronary heart disease: dietary links and pathogenesis. Public health nutrition, *4*(2b), 459-474.

[50] Yin, L., Zhong, G., & Liu, X. (2002). Research progress on nutritional characteristics, physiological function and medicinal value of buckwheat. Cereals & Oils, *33*(5), 32-34.

[51] Zhuang, W., Chen, H., Yang, M., Wang, J., Pandey, M. K., Zhang, C., ... & Garg, V. (2019). The genome of cultivated peanut provides insight into legume karyotypes, polyploid evolution and crop domestication. Nature genetics, *51*(5), 865-876.

[52] Gebremariam, M. M., Zarnkow, M., & Becker, T. (2014). Teff (Eragrostis tef) as a raw material for malting, brewing and manufacturing of gluten-free foods and beverages: a review. Journal of Food Science and Technology, 51(11), 2881-2895.

[53] Badejo, A. A., Olawoyin, B., Salawu, S. O., Fasuhanmi, O. S., Boligon, A. A., & Enujiugha, V. N. (2017). Antioxidative potentials and chromatographic analysis of beverages from blends of gluten-free acha (Digitaria exilis) and tigernut (Cyperus esculentus) extracts. Journal of Food Measurement and Characterization, *11*(4), 2094-2101.

[54] Sharma, M., Sangwan, R. S., Khatkar, B. S., & Singh, S. P. (2020). Development of a Prebiotic Oligosaccharide Rich Functional Beverage from Sweet Sorghum Stalk Biomass. Waste and Biomass Valorization, 1-12.

[55] Munekata, P. E. S., Rocchetti, G., Pateiro, M., Lucini, L., Domínguez, R., & Lorenzo, J. M. (2020). Addition of plant extracts to meat and meat products to extend shelf-life and health-promoting attributes: An overview. *Current Opinion in Food Science*.

[56] De Meo, B., Freeman, G., Marconi, O., Booer, C., Perretti, G., & Fantozzi, P. (2011). Behaviour of malted cereals and pseudo-cereals for gluten-free beer production. Journal of the Institute of Brewing, *117*(4), 541-546.

[57] Gumienna, M., & Górna, B. (2020). Gluten hypersensitivities and their impact on the production of gluten-free beer. European Food Research and Technology, 1-14.

[58] Nissen, L., Samaei, S. P., Babini, E., & Gianotti, A. (2020). Gluten free sourdough bread enriched with cricket flour for protein fortification: Antioxidant improvement and Volatilome characterization. Food Chemistry, 333, 127410.

[59] Weaver, K. N., & Herfarth, H. (2020). Gluten-free Diet in IBD: Time for a Recommendation? Molecular nutrition & food research, 1901274.

[60] Podeszwa, T. (2013). The use of pseudocereals for the production of gluten-free beer. Eng. Sci. Technol, 92-102.

[61] Rubio-Flores, M., & Serna-Saldivar, S. O. (2016). Technological and engineering trends for production of gluten-free beers. Food engineering reviews, *8*(4), 468-482.

[62] Food and Drug Administration (2015). Federal Register Food labelling: gluten-free labeling of fermented or hydrolyzed foods. Accessed on 11/18/2015 Docket No. FDA-2014-N-1021. https://www.regulations.gov Accessed 11/18/2015

[63] Kerpes, R., Fischer, S., & Becker, T. (2017). The production of gluten-free beer: Degradation of hordeins during malting and brewing and the application of modern process technology focusing on endogenous malt peptidases. Trends in Food Science & Technology, 67, 129-138.

[64] Yeo, H. Q., & Liu, S. Q. (2014). An overview of selected specialty beers: Developments, challenges and prospects. International journal of food science & technology, 49(7), 1607-1618.

[65] Mayer, H., Ceccaroni, D., Marconi, O., Sileoni, V., Perretti, G., & Fantozzi, P. (2016). Development of an all rice malt beer: A gluten free alternative. LWT-Food Science and Technology, *67*, 67-73.

[66] Hager, A. S., Taylor, J. P., Waters, D. M., & Arendt, E. K. (2014). Gluten free beer–A review. Trends in Food Science & Technology, *36*(1), 44-54.

[67] Sohrabvandi, S., Mortazavian, A. M., & Rezaei, K. (2012). Health-related aspects of beer: a review. International Journal of Food Properties, *15*(2), 350-373.

[68] Zweytik, G., & Berghofer, E. (2009). Production of gluten-free beer. In E. Gallagher (Ed.), Gluten-free food science and technology. Oxford, UK: Wiley-Blackwell.

[69] Ceppi, E. L. M., & Brenna, O. V. (2010). Brewing with rice malt—A gluten-free alternative. Journal of the Institute of Brewing, 116(3), 275-279.

[70] Gorgitano, M. T., & Sodano, V. (2019). Gluten-Free Products: From Dietary Necessity to Premium Price Extraction Tool. Nutrients, 11(9), 1997.

[71] Bogue, J., & Sorenson, D. (2008). 17 - The marketing of gluten-free cereal products. In E. K. Arendt & F. Dal Bello (Eds.), *Gluten-Free Cereal Products and Beverages* (pp. 393-411). Academic Press. https://doi.org/https://doi.org/10.1016/B978-012373739-7.50019-8

[72] Bagolin do Nascimento, A., Medeiros Rataichesck Fiates, G., dos Anjos, A., & Teixeira, E. (2014). Availability, cost and nutritional composition of gluten-free products. British Food Journal, *116*(12), 1842-1852. https://doi.org/10.1108/BFJ-05-2013-0131

[73] Lambert, K., & Ficken, C. (2016). Cost and affordability of a nutritionally balanced gluten-free diet: Is following a gluten-free diet affordable? [https://doi.org/10.1111/1747-0080.12171]. Nutrition & Dietetics, *73*(1), 36-42. https://doi.org/https://doi.org/10.1111/1747-0080.12171